**Week:** _____

### Monday  ___ / ___ / ___

| | Breakfast | | Lunch | | |
|---|---|---|---|---|---|
| | Before | After | Before | After | Bef |
| | | | | | |

### Tuesday  ___ / ___ / ___

| | Breakfast | | Lunch | | Dinner | | Bedtime | | Notes |
|---|---|---|---|---|---|---|---|---|---|
| | Before | After | Before | After | Before | After | Before | After | |
| | | | | | | | | | |

### Wednesday  ___ / ___ / ___

| | Breakfast | | Lunch | | Dinner | | Bedtime | | Notes |
|---|---|---|---|---|---|---|---|---|---|
| | Before | After | Before | After | Before | After | Before | After | |
| | | | | | | | | | |

### Thursday  ___ / ___ / ___

| | Breakfast | | Lunch | | Dinner | | Bedtime | | Notes |
|---|---|---|---|---|---|---|---|---|---|
| | Before | After | Before | After | Before | After | Before | After | |
| | | | | | | | | | |

### Friday  ___ / ___ / ___

| | Breakfast | | Lunch | | Dinner | | Bedtime | | Notes |
|---|---|---|---|---|---|---|---|---|---|
| | Before | After | Before | After | Before | After | Before | After | |
| | | | | | | | | | |

### Saturday  ___ / ___ / ___

| | Breakfast | | Lunch | | Dinner | | Bedtime | | Notes |
|---|---|---|---|---|---|---|---|---|---|
| | Before | After | Before | After | Before | After | Before | After | |
| | | | | | | | | | |

### Sunday  ___ / ___ / ___

| | Breakfast | | Lunch | | Dinner | | Bedtime | | Notes |
|---|---|---|---|---|---|---|---|---|---|
| | Before | After | Before | After | Before | After | Before | After | |
| | | | | | | | | | |

| Week: _____ | | | | | | | | | Weight: _____ |

| Monday | Breakfast | | Lunch | | Dinner | | Bedtime | | Notes |
|---|---|---|---|---|---|---|---|---|---|
| | Before | After | Before | After | Before | After | Before | After | |
| __/__/__ | | | | | | | | | |

| Tuesday | Breakfast | | Lunch | | Dinner | | Bedtime | | Notes |
|---|---|---|---|---|---|---|---|---|---|
| | Before | After | Before | After | Before | After | Before | After | |
| __/__/__ | | | | | | | | | |

| Wednesday | Breakfast | | Lunch | | Dinner | | Bedtime | | Notes |
|---|---|---|---|---|---|---|---|---|---|
| | Before | After | Before | After | Before | After | Before | After | |
| __/__/__ | | | | | | | | | |

| Thursday | Breakfast | | Lunch | | Dinner | | Bedtime | | Notes |
|---|---|---|---|---|---|---|---|---|---|
| | Before | After | Before | After | Before | After | Before | After | |
| __/__/__ | | | | | | | | | |

| Friday | Breakfast | | Lunch | | Dinner | | Bedtime | | Notes |
|---|---|---|---|---|---|---|---|---|---|
| | Before | After | Before | After | Before | After | Before | After | |
| __/__/__ | | | | | | | | | |

| Saturday | Breakfast | | Lunch | | Dinner | | Bedtime | | Notes |
|---|---|---|---|---|---|---|---|---|---|
| | Before | After | Before | After | Before | After | Before | After | |
| __/__/__ | | | | | | | | | |

| Sunday | Breakfast | | Lunch | | Dinner | | Bedtime | | Notes |
|---|---|---|---|---|---|---|---|---|---|
| | Before | After | Before | After | Before | After | Before | After | |
| __/__/__ | | | | | | | | | |

| Week: _____ | | | | | | | | | Weight: _____ |

| Monday | Breakfast | | Lunch | | Dinner | | Bedtime | | Notes |
|---|---|---|---|---|---|---|---|---|---|
| | Before | After | Before | After | Before | After | Before | After | |
| __ / __ / __ | | | | | | | | | |

| Tuesday | Breakfast | | Lunch | | Dinner | | Bedtime | | Notes |
|---|---|---|---|---|---|---|---|---|---|
| | Before | After | Before | After | Before | After | Before | After | |
| __ / __ / __ | | | | | | | | | |

| Wednesday | Breakfast | | Lunch | | Dinner | | Bedtime | | Notes |
|---|---|---|---|---|---|---|---|---|---|
| | Before | After | Before | After | Before | After | Before | After | |
| __ / __ / __ | | | | | | | | | |

| Thursday | Breakfast | | Lunch | | Dinner | | Bedtime | | Notes |
|---|---|---|---|---|---|---|---|---|---|
| | Before | After | Before | After | Before | After | Before | After | |
| __ / __ / __ | | | | | | | | | |

| Friday | Breakfast | | Lunch | | Dinner | | Bedtime | | Notes |
|---|---|---|---|---|---|---|---|---|---|
| | Before | After | Before | After | Before | After | Before | After | |
| __ / __ / __ | | | | | | | | | |

| Saturday | Breakfast | | Lunch | | Dinner | | Bedtime | | Notes |
|---|---|---|---|---|---|---|---|---|---|
| | Before | After | Before | After | Before | After | Before | After | |
| __ / __ / __ | | | | | | | | | |

| Sunday | Breakfast | | Lunch | | Dinner | | Bedtime | | Notes |
|---|---|---|---|---|---|---|---|---|---|
| | Before | After | Before | After | Before | After | Before | After | |
| __ / __ / __ | | | | | | | | | |

| Week: _____ | | | | | | | | | Weight: _____ |

| Monday | Breakfast | | Lunch | | Dinner | | Bedtime | | Notes |
|---|---|---|---|---|---|---|---|---|---|
| | Before | After | Before | After | Before | After | Before | After | |
| __/__/__ | | | | | | | | | |

| Tuesday | Breakfast | | Lunch | | Dinner | | Bedtime | | Notes |
|---|---|---|---|---|---|---|---|---|---|
| | Before | After | Before | After | Before | After | Before | After | |
| __/__/__ | | | | | | | | | |

| Wednesday | Breakfast | | Lunch | | Dinner | | Bedtime | | Notes |
|---|---|---|---|---|---|---|---|---|---|
| | Before | After | Before | After | Before | After | Before | After | |
| __/__/__ | | | | | | | | | |

| Thursday | Breakfast | | Lunch | | Dinner | | Bedtime | | Notes |
|---|---|---|---|---|---|---|---|---|---|
| | Before | After | Before | After | Before | After | Before | After | |
| __/__/__ | | | | | | | | | |

| Friday | Breakfast | | Lunch | | Dinner | | Bedtime | | Notes |
|---|---|---|---|---|---|---|---|---|---|
| | Before | After | Before | After | Before | After | Before | After | |
| __/__/__ | | | | | | | | | |

| Saturday | Breakfast | | Lunch | | Dinner | | Bedtime | | Notes |
|---|---|---|---|---|---|---|---|---|---|
| | Before | After | Before | After | Before | After | Before | After | |
| __/__/__ | | | | | | | | | |

| Sunday | Breakfast | | Lunch | | Dinner | | Bedtime | | Notes |
|---|---|---|---|---|---|---|---|---|---|
| | Before | After | Before | After | Before | After | Before | After | |
| __/__/__ | | | | | | | | | |

| Week: _____ | | | | | | | | | Weight: _____ |

| Monday | Breakfast | | Lunch | | Dinner | | Bedtime | | Notes |
|---|---|---|---|---|---|---|---|---|---|
| | Before | After | Before | After | Before | After | Before | After | |
| __ / __ / __ | | | | | | | | | |

| Tuesday | Breakfast | | Lunch | | Dinner | | Bedtime | | Notes |
|---|---|---|---|---|---|---|---|---|---|
| | Before | After | Before | After | Before | After | Before | After | |
| __ / __ / __ | | | | | | | | | |

| Wednesday | Breakfast | | Lunch | | Dinner | | Bedtime | | Notes |
|---|---|---|---|---|---|---|---|---|---|
| | Before | After | Before | After | Before | After | Before | After | |
| __ / __ / __ | | | | | | | | | |

| Thursday | Breakfast | | Lunch | | Dinner | | Bedtime | | Notes |
|---|---|---|---|---|---|---|---|---|---|
| | Before | After | Before | After | Before | After | Before | After | |
| __ / __ / __ | | | | | | | | | |

| Friday | Breakfast | | Lunch | | Dinner | | Bedtime | | Notes |
|---|---|---|---|---|---|---|---|---|---|
| | Before | After | Before | After | Before | After | Before | After | |
| __ / __ / __ | | | | | | | | | |

| Saturday | Breakfast | | Lunch | | Dinner | | Bedtime | | Notes |
|---|---|---|---|---|---|---|---|---|---|
| | Before | After | Before | After | Before | After | Before | After | |
| __ / __ / __ | | | | | | | | | |

| Sunday | Breakfast | | Lunch | | Dinner | | Bedtime | | Notes |
|---|---|---|---|---|---|---|---|---|---|
| | Before | After | Before | After | Before | After | Before | After | |
| __ / __ / __ | | | | | | | | | |

| Week: _____ | | | | | | | | | Weight: _____ |

| Monday | Breakfast | | Lunch | | Dinner | | Bedtime | | Notes |
|---|---|---|---|---|---|---|---|---|---|
| | Before | After | Before | After | Before | After | Before | After | |
| __/__/__ | | | | | | | | | |

| Tuesday | Breakfast | | Lunch | | Dinner | | Bedtime | | Notes |
|---|---|---|---|---|---|---|---|---|---|
| | Before | After | Before | After | Before | After | Before | After | |
| __/__/__ | | | | | | | | | |

| Wednesday | Breakfast | | Lunch | | Dinner | | Bedtime | | Notes |
|---|---|---|---|---|---|---|---|---|---|
| | Before | After | Before | After | Before | After | Before | After | |
| __/__/__ | | | | | | | | | |

| Thursday | Breakfast | | Lunch | | Dinner | | Bedtime | | Notes |
|---|---|---|---|---|---|---|---|---|---|
| | Before | After | Before | After | Before | After | Before | After | |
| __/__/__ | | | | | | | | | |

| Friday | Breakfast | | Lunch | | Dinner | | Bedtime | | Notes |
|---|---|---|---|---|---|---|---|---|---|
| | Before | After | Before | After | Before | After | Before | After | |
| __/__/__ | | | | | | | | | |

| Saturday | Breakfast | | Lunch | | Dinner | | Bedtime | | Notes |
|---|---|---|---|---|---|---|---|---|---|
| | Before | After | Before | After | Before | After | Before | After | |
| __/__/__ | | | | | | | | | |

| Sunday | Breakfast | | Lunch | | Dinner | | Bedtime | | Notes |
|---|---|---|---|---|---|---|---|---|---|
| | Before | After | Before | After | Before | After | Before | After | |
| __/__/__ | | | | | | | | | |

| Week: _____ | | | | | | | | | Weight: _____ |

| Monday | Breakfast | | Lunch | | Dinner | | Bedtime | | Notes |
|---|---|---|---|---|---|---|---|---|---|
| | Before | After | Before | After | Before | After | Before | After | |
| __ / __ / __ | | | | | | | | | |

| Tuesday | Breakfast | | Lunch | | Dinner | | Bedtime | | Notes |
|---|---|---|---|---|---|---|---|---|---|
| | Before | After | Before | After | Before | After | Before | After | |
| __ / __ / __ | | | | | | | | | |

| Wednesday | Breakfast | | Lunch | | Dinner | | Bedtime | | Notes |
|---|---|---|---|---|---|---|---|---|---|
| | Before | After | Before | After | Before | After | Before | After | |
| __ / __ / __ | | | | | | | | | |

| Thursday | Breakfast | | Lunch | | Dinner | | Bedtime | | Notes |
|---|---|---|---|---|---|---|---|---|---|
| | Before | After | Before | After | Before | After | Before | After | |
| __ / __ / __ | | | | | | | | | |

| Friday | Breakfast | | Lunch | | Dinner | | Bedtime | | Notes |
|---|---|---|---|---|---|---|---|---|---|
| | Before | After | Before | After | Before | After | Before | After | |
| __ / __ / __ | | | | | | | | | |

| Saturday | Breakfast | | Lunch | | Dinner | | Bedtime | | Notes |
|---|---|---|---|---|---|---|---|---|---|
| | Before | After | Before | After | Before | After | Before | After | |
| __ / __ / __ | | | | | | | | | |

| Sunday | Breakfast | | Lunch | | Dinner | | Bedtime | | Notes |
|---|---|---|---|---|---|---|---|---|---|
| | Before | After | Before | After | Before | After | Before | After | |
| __ / __ / __ | | | | | | | | | |

| Week: _____ | | | | | | | | | Weight: _____ |

| Monday | Breakfast | | Lunch | | Dinner | | Bedtime | | Notes |
|---|---|---|---|---|---|---|---|---|---|
| | Before | After | Before | After | Before | After | Before | After | |
| __/__/__ | | | | | | | | | |

| Tuesday | Breakfast | | Lunch | | Dinner | | Bedtime | | Notes |
|---|---|---|---|---|---|---|---|---|---|
| | Before | After | Before | After | Before | After | Before | After | |
| __/__/__ | | | | | | | | | |

| Wednesday | Breakfast | | Lunch | | Dinner | | Bedtime | | Notes |
|---|---|---|---|---|---|---|---|---|---|
| | Before | After | Before | After | Before | After | Before | After | |
| __/__/__ | | | | | | | | | |

| Thursday | Breakfast | | Lunch | | Dinner | | Bedtime | | Notes |
|---|---|---|---|---|---|---|---|---|---|
| | Before | After | Before | After | Before | After | Before | After | |
| __/__/__ | | | | | | | | | |

| Friday | Breakfast | | Lunch | | Dinner | | Bedtime | | Notes |
|---|---|---|---|---|---|---|---|---|---|
| | Before | After | Before | After | Before | After | Before | After | |
| __/__/__ | | | | | | | | | |

| Saturday | Breakfast | | Lunch | | Dinner | | Bedtime | | Notes |
|---|---|---|---|---|---|---|---|---|---|
| | Before | After | Before | After | Before | After | Before | After | |
| __/__/__ | | | | | | | | | |

| Sunday | Breakfast | | Lunch | | Dinner | | Bedtime | | Notes |
|---|---|---|---|---|---|---|---|---|---|
| | Before | After | Before | After | Before | After | Before | After | |
| __/__/__ | | | | | | | | | |

| Week: _____ | | | | | | | | | Weight: _____ |

| Monday | Breakfast | | Lunch | | Dinner | | Bedtime | | Notes |
|---|---|---|---|---|---|---|---|---|---|
| | Before | After | Before | After | Before | After | Before | After | |
| __ / __ / __ | | | | | | | | | |

| Tuesday | Breakfast | | Lunch | | Dinner | | Bedtime | | Notes |
|---|---|---|---|---|---|---|---|---|---|
| | Before | After | Before | After | Before | After | Before | After | |
| __ / __ / __ | | | | | | | | | |

| Wednesday | Breakfast | | Lunch | | Dinner | | Bedtime | | Notes |
|---|---|---|---|---|---|---|---|---|---|
| | Before | After | Before | After | Before | After | Before | After | |
| __ / __ / __ | | | | | | | | | |

| Thursday | Breakfast | | Lunch | | Dinner | | Bedtime | | Notes |
|---|---|---|---|---|---|---|---|---|---|
| | Before | After | Before | After | Before | After | Before | After | |
| __ / __ / __ | | | | | | | | | |

| Friday | Breakfast | | Lunch | | Dinner | | Bedtime | | Notes |
|---|---|---|---|---|---|---|---|---|---|
| | Before | After | Before | After | Before | After | Before | After | |
| __ / __ / __ | | | | | | | | | |

| Saturday | Breakfast | | Lunch | | Dinner | | Bedtime | | Notes |
|---|---|---|---|---|---|---|---|---|---|
| | Before | After | Before | After | Before | After | Before | After | |
| __ / __ / __ | | | | | | | | | |

| Sunday | Breakfast | | Lunch | | Dinner | | Bedtime | | Notes |
|---|---|---|---|---|---|---|---|---|---|
| | Before | After | Before | After | Before | After | Before | After | |
| __ / __ / __ | | | | | | | | | |

| Week: _____ | | | | | | | | | Weight: _____ |
|---|---|---|---|---|---|---|---|---|---|

| Monday | Breakfast | | Lunch | | Dinner | | Bedtime | | Notes |
|---|---|---|---|---|---|---|---|---|---|
| | Before | After | Before | After | Before | After | Before | After | |
| __/__/__ | | | | | | | | | |

| Tuesday | Breakfast | | Lunch | | Dinner | | Bedtime | | Notes |
|---|---|---|---|---|---|---|---|---|---|
| | Before | After | Before | After | Before | After | Before | After | |
| __/__/__ | | | | | | | | | |

| Wednesday | Breakfast | | Lunch | | Dinner | | Bedtime | | Notes |
|---|---|---|---|---|---|---|---|---|---|
| | Before | After | Before | After | Before | After | Before | After | |
| __/__/__ | | | | | | | | | |

| Thursday | Breakfast | | Lunch | | Dinner | | Bedtime | | Notes |
|---|---|---|---|---|---|---|---|---|---|
| | Before | After | Before | After | Before | After | Before | After | |
| __/__/__ | | | | | | | | | |

| Friday | Breakfast | | Lunch | | Dinner | | Bedtime | | Notes |
|---|---|---|---|---|---|---|---|---|---|
| | Before | After | Before | After | Before | After | Before | After | |
| __/__/__ | | | | | | | | | |

| Saturday | Breakfast | | Lunch | | Dinner | | Bedtime | | Notes |
|---|---|---|---|---|---|---|---|---|---|
| | Before | After | Before | After | Before | After | Before | After | |
| __/__/__ | | | | | | | | | |

| Sunday | Breakfast | | Lunch | | Dinner | | Bedtime | | Notes |
|---|---|---|---|---|---|---|---|---|---|
| | Before | After | Before | After | Before | After | Before | After | |
| __/__/__ | | | | | | | | | |

| Week: _____ | | | | | | | | | Weight: _____ |
|---|---|---|---|---|---|---|---|---|---|

| Monday | Breakfast | | Lunch | | Dinner | | Bedtime | | Notes |
|---|---|---|---|---|---|---|---|---|---|
| | Before | After | Before | After | Before | After | Before | After | |
| __ / __ / __ | | | | | | | | | |

| Tuesday | Breakfast | | Lunch | | Dinner | | Bedtime | | Notes |
|---|---|---|---|---|---|---|---|---|---|
| | Before | After | Before | After | Before | After | Before | After | |
| __ / __ / __ | | | | | | | | | |

| Wednesday | Breakfast | | Lunch | | Dinner | | Bedtime | | Notes |
|---|---|---|---|---|---|---|---|---|---|
| | Before | After | Before | After | Before | After | Before | After | |
| __ / __ / __ | | | | | | | | | |

| Thursday | Breakfast | | Lunch | | Dinner | | Bedtime | | Notes |
|---|---|---|---|---|---|---|---|---|---|
| | Before | After | Before | After | Before | After | Before | After | |
| __ / __ / __ | | | | | | | | | |

| Friday | Breakfast | | Lunch | | Dinner | | Bedtime | | Notes |
|---|---|---|---|---|---|---|---|---|---|
| | Before | After | Before | After | Before | After | Before | After | |
| __ / __ / __ | | | | | | | | | |

| Saturday | Breakfast | | Lunch | | Dinner | | Bedtime | | Notes |
|---|---|---|---|---|---|---|---|---|---|
| | Before | After | Before | After | Before | After | Before | After | |
| __ / __ / __ | | | | | | | | | |

| Sunday | Breakfast | | Lunch | | Dinner | | Bedtime | | Notes |
|---|---|---|---|---|---|---|---|---|---|
| | Before | After | Before | After | Before | After | Before | After | |
| __ / __ / __ | | | | | | | | | |

| Week: _____ | | | | | | | | | Weight: _____ |

| Monday | Breakfast | | Lunch | | Dinner | | Bedtime | | Notes |
|---|---|---|---|---|---|---|---|---|---|
| | Before | After | Before | After | Before | After | Before | After | |
| __/__/__ | | | | | | | | | |

| Tuesday | Breakfast | | Lunch | | Dinner | | Bedtime | | Notes |
|---|---|---|---|---|---|---|---|---|---|
| | Before | After | Before | After | Before | After | Before | After | |
| __/__/__ | | | | | | | | | |

| Wednesday | Breakfast | | Lunch | | Dinner | | Bedtime | | Notes |
|---|---|---|---|---|---|---|---|---|---|
| | Before | After | Before | After | Before | After | Before | After | |
| __/__/__ | | | | | | | | | |

| Thursday | Breakfast | | Lunch | | Dinner | | Bedtime | | Notes |
|---|---|---|---|---|---|---|---|---|---|
| | Before | After | Before | After | Before | After | Before | After | |
| __/__/__ | | | | | | | | | |

| Friday | Breakfast | | Lunch | | Dinner | | Bedtime | | Notes |
|---|---|---|---|---|---|---|---|---|---|
| | Before | After | Before | After | Before | After | Before | After | |
| __/__/__ | | | | | | | | | |

| Saturday | Breakfast | | Lunch | | Dinner | | Bedtime | | Notes |
|---|---|---|---|---|---|---|---|---|---|
| | Before | After | Before | After | Before | After | Before | After | |
| __/__/__ | | | | | | | | | |

| Sunday | Breakfast | | Lunch | | Dinner | | Bedtime | | Notes |
|---|---|---|---|---|---|---|---|---|---|
| | Before | After | Before | After | Before | After | Before | After | |
| __/__/__ | | | | | | | | | |

| Week: _____ | | | | | | | | | Weight: _____ |

| Monday | Breakfast | | Lunch | | Dinner | | Bedtime | | Notes |
|---|---|---|---|---|---|---|---|---|---|
| | Before | After | Before | After | Before | After | Before | After | |
| __/__/__ | | | | | | | | | |

| Tuesday | Breakfast | | Lunch | | Dinner | | Bedtime | | Notes |
|---|---|---|---|---|---|---|---|---|---|
| | Before | After | Before | After | Before | After | Before | After | |
| __/__/__ | | | | | | | | | |

| Wednesday | Breakfast | | Lunch | | Dinner | | Bedtime | | Notes |
|---|---|---|---|---|---|---|---|---|---|
| | Before | After | Before | After | Before | After | Before | After | |
| __/__/__ | | | | | | | | | |

| Thursday | Breakfast | | Lunch | | Dinner | | Bedtime | | Notes |
|---|---|---|---|---|---|---|---|---|---|
| | Before | After | Before | After | Before | After | Before | After | |
| __/__/__ | | | | | | | | | |

| Friday | Breakfast | | Lunch | | Dinner | | Bedtime | | Notes |
|---|---|---|---|---|---|---|---|---|---|
| | Before | After | Before | After | Before | After | Before | After | |
| __/__/__ | | | | | | | | | |

| Saturday | Breakfast | | Lunch | | Dinner | | Bedtime | | Notes |
|---|---|---|---|---|---|---|---|---|---|
| | Before | After | Before | After | Before | After | Before | After | |
| __/__/__ | | | | | | | | | |

| Sunday | Breakfast | | Lunch | | Dinner | | Bedtime | | Notes |
|---|---|---|---|---|---|---|---|---|---|
| | Before | After | Before | After | Before | After | Before | After | |
| __/__/__ | | | | | | | | | |

**Week:** _____  **Weight:** _____

| Monday | Breakfast | | Lunch | | Dinner | | Bedtime | | Notes |
|---|---|---|---|---|---|---|---|---|---|
| | Before | After | Before | After | Before | After | Before | After | |
| \_\_ / \_\_ / \_\_ | | | | | | | | | |

| Tuesday | Breakfast | | Lunch | | Dinner | | Bedtime | | Notes |
|---|---|---|---|---|---|---|---|---|---|
| | Before | After | Before | After | Before | After | Before | After | |
| \_\_ / \_\_ / \_\_ | | | | | | | | | |

| Wednesday | Breakfast | | Lunch | | Dinner | | Bedtime | | Notes |
|---|---|---|---|---|---|---|---|---|---|
| | Before | After | Before | After | Before | After | Before | After | |
| \_\_ / \_\_ / \_\_ | | | | | | | | | |

| Thursday | Breakfast | | Lunch | | Dinner | | Bedtime | | Notes |
|---|---|---|---|---|---|---|---|---|---|
| | Before | After | Before | After | Before | After | Before | After | |
| \_\_ / \_\_ / \_\_ | | | | | | | | | |

| Friday | Breakfast | | Lunch | | Dinner | | Bedtime | | Notes |
|---|---|---|---|---|---|---|---|---|---|
| | Before | After | Before | After | Before | After | Before | After | |
| \_\_ / \_\_ / \_\_ | | | | | | | | | |

| Saturday | Breakfast | | Lunch | | Dinner | | Bedtime | | Notes |
|---|---|---|---|---|---|---|---|---|---|
| | Before | After | Before | After | Before | After | Before | After | |
| \_\_ / \_\_ / \_\_ | | | | | | | | | |

| Sunday | Breakfast | | Lunch | | Dinner | | Bedtime | | Notes |
|---|---|---|---|---|---|---|---|---|---|
| | Before | After | Before | After | Before | After | Before | After | |
| \_\_ / \_\_ / \_\_ | | | | | | | | | |

| Monday | Breakfast | | Lunch | | Dinner | | Bedtime | | Notes |
|---|---|---|---|---|---|---|---|---|---|
| | Before | After | Before | After | Before | After | Before | After | |
| __ / __ / __ | | | | | | | | | |

| Tuesday | Breakfast | | Lunch | | Dinner | | Bedtime | | Notes |
|---|---|---|---|---|---|---|---|---|---|
| | Before | After | Before | After | Before | After | Before | After | |
| __ / __ / __ | | | | | | | | | |

| Wednesday | Breakfast | | Lunch | | Dinner | | Bedtime | | Notes |
|---|---|---|---|---|---|---|---|---|---|
| | Before | After | Before | After | Before | After | Before | After | |
| __ / __ / __ | | | | | | | | | |

| Thursday | Breakfast | | Lunch | | Dinner | | Bedtime | | Notes |
|---|---|---|---|---|---|---|---|---|---|
| | Before | After | Before | After | Before | After | Before | After | |
| __ / __ / __ | | | | | | | | | |

| Friday | Breakfast | | Lunch | | Dinner | | Bedtime | | Notes |
|---|---|---|---|---|---|---|---|---|---|
| | Before | After | Before | After | Before | After | Before | After | |
| __ / __ / __ | | | | | | | | | |

| Saturday | Breakfast | | Lunch | | Dinner | | Bedtime | | Notes |
|---|---|---|---|---|---|---|---|---|---|
| | Before | After | Before | After | Before | After | Before | After | |
| __ / __ / __ | | | | | | | | | |

| Sunday | Breakfast | | Lunch | | Dinner | | Bedtime | | Notes |
|---|---|---|---|---|---|---|---|---|---|
| | Before | After | Before | After | Before | After | Before | After | |
| __ / __ / __ | | | | | | | | | |

| Week: _____ | | | | | | | | | Weight: _____ |
|---|---|---|---|---|---|---|---|---|---|

| Monday | Breakfast | | Lunch | | Dinner | | Bedtime | | Notes |
|---|---|---|---|---|---|---|---|---|---|
| | Before | After | Before | After | Before | After | Before | After | |
| __ / __ / __ | | | | | | | | | |

| Tuesday | Breakfast | | Lunch | | Dinner | | Bedtime | | Notes |
|---|---|---|---|---|---|---|---|---|---|
| | Before | After | Before | After | Before | After | Before | After | |
| __ / __ / __ | | | | | | | | | |

| Wednesday | Breakfast | | Lunch | | Dinner | | Bedtime | | Notes |
|---|---|---|---|---|---|---|---|---|---|
| | Before | After | Before | After | Before | After | Before | After | |
| __ / __ / __ | | | | | | | | | |

| Thursday | Breakfast | | Lunch | | Dinner | | Bedtime | | Notes |
|---|---|---|---|---|---|---|---|---|---|
| | Before | After | Before | After | Before | After | Before | After | |
| __ / __ / __ | | | | | | | | | |

| Friday | Breakfast | | Lunch | | Dinner | | Bedtime | | Notes |
|---|---|---|---|---|---|---|---|---|---|
| | Before | After | Before | After | Before | After | Before | After | |
| __ / __ / __ | | | | | | | | | |

| Saturday | Breakfast | | Lunch | | Dinner | | Bedtime | | Notes |
|---|---|---|---|---|---|---|---|---|---|
| | Before | After | Before | After | Before | After | Before | After | |
| __ / __ / __ | | | | | | | | | |

| Sunday | Breakfast | | Lunch | | Dinner | | Bedtime | | Notes |
|---|---|---|---|---|---|---|---|---|---|
| | Before | After | Before | After | Before | After | Before | After | |
| __ / __ / __ | | | | | | | | | |

| Week: _____ | | | | | | | | | Weight: _____ |

| Monday | Breakfast | | Lunch | | Dinner | | Bedtime | | Notes |
|---|---|---|---|---|---|---|---|---|---|
| | Before | After | Before | After | Before | After | Before | After | |
| __/__/__ | | | | | | | | | |

| Tuesday | Breakfast | | Lunch | | Dinner | | Bedtime | | Notes |
|---|---|---|---|---|---|---|---|---|---|
| | Before | After | Before | After | Before | After | Before | After | |
| __/__/__ | | | | | | | | | |

| Wednesday | Breakfast | | Lunch | | Dinner | | Bedtime | | Notes |
|---|---|---|---|---|---|---|---|---|---|
| | Before | After | Before | After | Before | After | Before | After | |
| __/__/__ | | | | | | | | | |

| Thursday | Breakfast | | Lunch | | Dinner | | Bedtime | | Notes |
|---|---|---|---|---|---|---|---|---|---|
| | Before | After | Before | After | Before | After | Before | After | |
| __/__/__ | | | | | | | | | |

| Friday | Breakfast | | Lunch | | Dinner | | Bedtime | | Notes |
|---|---|---|---|---|---|---|---|---|---|
| | Before | After | Before | After | Before | After | Before | After | |
| __/__/__ | | | | | | | | | |

| Saturday | Breakfast | | Lunch | | Dinner | | Bedtime | | Notes |
|---|---|---|---|---|---|---|---|---|---|
| | Before | After | Before | After | Before | After | Before | After | |
| __/__/__ | | | | | | | | | |

| Sunday | Breakfast | | Lunch | | Dinner | | Bedtime | | Notes |
|---|---|---|---|---|---|---|---|---|---|
| | Before | After | Before | After | Before | After | Before | After | |
| __/__/__ | | | | | | | | | |

| Week: _____ | | | | | | | | | Weight: _____ |

| Monday | Breakfast | | Lunch | | Dinner | | Bedtime | | Notes |
|---|---|---|---|---|---|---|---|---|---|
| | Before | After | Before | After | Before | After | Before | After | |
| __ / __ / __ | | | | | | | | | |

| Tuesday | Breakfast | | Lunch | | Dinner | | Bedtime | | Notes |
|---|---|---|---|---|---|---|---|---|---|
| | Before | After | Before | After | Before | After | Before | After | |
| __ / __ / __ | | | | | | | | | |

| Wednesday | Breakfast | | Lunch | | Dinner | | Bedtime | | Notes |
|---|---|---|---|---|---|---|---|---|---|
| | Before | After | Before | After | Before | After | Before | After | |
| __ / __ / __ | | | | | | | | | |

| Thursday | Breakfast | | Lunch | | Dinner | | Bedtime | | Notes |
|---|---|---|---|---|---|---|---|---|---|
| | Before | After | Before | After | Before | After | Before | After | |
| __ / __ / __ | | | | | | | | | |

| Friday | Breakfast | | Lunch | | Dinner | | Bedtime | | Notes |
|---|---|---|---|---|---|---|---|---|---|
| | Before | After | Before | After | Before | After | Before | After | |
| __ / __ / __ | | | | | | | | | |

| Saturday | Breakfast | | Lunch | | Dinner | | Bedtime | | Notes |
|---|---|---|---|---|---|---|---|---|---|
| | Before | After | Before | After | Before | After | Before | After | |
| __ / __ / __ | | | | | | | | | |

| Sunday | Breakfast | | Lunch | | Dinner | | Bedtime | | Notes |
|---|---|---|---|---|---|---|---|---|---|
| | Before | After | Before | After | Before | After | Before | After | |
| __ / __ / __ | | | | | | | | | |

<table>
<tr><td>Week: _____</td><td colspan="9"></td><td>Weight: _____</td></tr>
</table>

| Monday | Breakfast | | Lunch | | Dinner | | Bedtime | | Notes |
|---|---|---|---|---|---|---|---|---|---|
| | Before | After | Before | After | Before | After | Before | After | |
| __ / __ / __ | | | | | | | | | |

| Tuesday | Breakfast | | Lunch | | Dinner | | Bedtime | | Notes |
|---|---|---|---|---|---|---|---|---|---|
| | Before | After | Before | After | Before | After | Before | After | |
| __ / __ / __ | | | | | | | | | |

| Wednesday | Breakfast | | Lunch | | Dinner | | Bedtime | | Notes |
|---|---|---|---|---|---|---|---|---|---|
| | Before | After | Before | After | Before | After | Before | After | |
| __ / __ / __ | | | | | | | | | |

| Thursday | Breakfast | | Lunch | | Dinner | | Bedtime | | Notes |
|---|---|---|---|---|---|---|---|---|---|
| | Before | After | Before | After | Before | After | Before | After | |
| __ / __ / __ | | | | | | | | | |

| Friday | Breakfast | | Lunch | | Dinner | | Bedtime | | Notes |
|---|---|---|---|---|---|---|---|---|---|
| | Before | After | Before | After | Before | After | Before | After | |
| __ / __ / __ | | | | | | | | | |

| Saturday | Breakfast | | Lunch | | Dinner | | Bedtime | | Notes |
|---|---|---|---|---|---|---|---|---|---|
| | Before | After | Before | After | Before | After | Before | After | |
| __ / __ / __ | | | | | | | | | |

| Sunday | Breakfast | | Lunch | | Dinner | | Bedtime | | Notes |
|---|---|---|---|---|---|---|---|---|---|
| | Before | After | Before | After | Before | After | Before | After | |
| __ / __ / __ | | | | | | | | | |

| Week: _____ | | | | | | | | | Weight: _____ |

| Monday | Breakfast | | Lunch | | Dinner | | Bedtime | | Notes |
|---|---|---|---|---|---|---|---|---|---|
| | Before | After | Before | After | Before | After | Before | After | |
| __ / __ / __ | | | | | | | | | |

| Tuesday | Breakfast | | Lunch | | Dinner | | Bedtime | | Notes |
|---|---|---|---|---|---|---|---|---|---|
| | Before | After | Before | After | Before | After | Before | After | |
| __ / __ / __ | | | | | | | | | |

| Wednesday | Breakfast | | Lunch | | Dinner | | Bedtime | | Notes |
|---|---|---|---|---|---|---|---|---|---|
| | Before | After | Before | After | Before | After | Before | After | |
| __ / __ / __ | | | | | | | | | |

| Thursday | Breakfast | | Lunch | | Dinner | | Bedtime | | Notes |
|---|---|---|---|---|---|---|---|---|---|
| | Before | After | Before | After | Before | After | Before | After | |
| __ / __ / __ | | | | | | | | | |

| Friday | Breakfast | | Lunch | | Dinner | | Bedtime | | Notes |
|---|---|---|---|---|---|---|---|---|---|
| | Before | After | Before | After | Before | After | Before | After | |
| __ / __ / __ | | | | | | | | | |

| Saturday | Breakfast | | Lunch | | Dinner | | Bedtime | | Notes |
|---|---|---|---|---|---|---|---|---|---|
| | Before | After | Before | After | Before | After | Before | After | |
| __ / __ / __ | | | | | | | | | |

| Sunday | Breakfast | | Lunch | | Dinner | | Bedtime | | Notes |
|---|---|---|---|---|---|---|---|---|---|
| | Before | After | Before | After | Before | After | Before | After | |
| __ / __ / __ | | | | | | | | | |

| Week: _____ | | | | | | | | | Weight: _____ |
|---|---|---|---|---|---|---|---|---|---|

| Monday | Breakfast | | Lunch | | Dinner | | Bedtime | | Notes |
|---|---|---|---|---|---|---|---|---|---|
| | Before | After | Before | After | Before | After | Before | After | |
| __ / __ / __ | | | | | | | | | |

| Tuesday | Breakfast | | Lunch | | Dinner | | Bedtime | | Notes |
|---|---|---|---|---|---|---|---|---|---|
| | Before | After | Before | After | Before | After | Before | After | |
| __ / __ / __ | | | | | | | | | |

| Wednesday | Breakfast | | Lunch | | Dinner | | Bedtime | | Notes |
|---|---|---|---|---|---|---|---|---|---|
| | Before | After | Before | After | Before | After | Before | After | |
| __ / __ / __ | | | | | | | | | |

| Thursday | Breakfast | | Lunch | | Dinner | | Bedtime | | Notes |
|---|---|---|---|---|---|---|---|---|---|
| | Before | After | Before | After | Before | After | Before | After | |
| __ / __ / __ | | | | | | | | | |

| Friday | Breakfast | | Lunch | | Dinner | | Bedtime | | Notes |
|---|---|---|---|---|---|---|---|---|---|
| | Before | After | Before | After | Before | After | Before | After | |
| __ / __ / __ | | | | | | | | | |

| Saturday | Breakfast | | Lunch | | Dinner | | Bedtime | | Notes |
|---|---|---|---|---|---|---|---|---|---|
| | Before | After | Before | After | Before | After | Before | After | |
| __ / __ / __ | | | | | | | | | |

| Sunday | Breakfast | | Lunch | | Dinner | | Bedtime | | Notes |
|---|---|---|---|---|---|---|---|---|---|
| | Before | After | Before | After | Before | After | Before | After | |
| __ / __ / __ | | | | | | | | | |

| Week: _____ | | | | | | | | | Weight: _____ |

| Monday | Breakfast | | Lunch | | Dinner | | Bedtime | | Notes |
|---|---|---|---|---|---|---|---|---|---|
| | Before | After | Before | After | Before | After | Before | After | |
| \_\_ / \_\_ / \_\_ | | | | | | | | | |

| Tuesday | Breakfast | | Lunch | | Dinner | | Bedtime | | Notes |
|---|---|---|---|---|---|---|---|---|---|
| | Before | After | Before | After | Before | After | Before | After | |
| \_\_ / \_\_ / \_\_ | | | | | | | | | |

| Wednesday | Breakfast | | Lunch | | Dinner | | Bedtime | | Notes |
|---|---|---|---|---|---|---|---|---|---|
| | Before | After | Before | After | Before | After | Before | After | |
| \_\_ / \_\_ / \_\_ | | | | | | | | | |

| Thursday | Breakfast | | Lunch | | Dinner | | Bedtime | | Notes |
|---|---|---|---|---|---|---|---|---|---|
| | Before | After | Before | After | Before | After | Before | After | |
| \_\_ / \_\_ / \_\_ | | | | | | | | | |

| Friday | Breakfast | | Lunch | | Dinner | | Bedtime | | Notes |
|---|---|---|---|---|---|---|---|---|---|
| | Before | After | Before | After | Before | After | Before | After | |
| \_\_ / \_\_ / \_\_ | | | | | | | | | |

| Saturday | Breakfast | | Lunch | | Dinner | | Bedtime | | Notes |
|---|---|---|---|---|---|---|---|---|---|
| | Before | After | Before | After | Before | After | Before | After | |
| \_\_ / \_\_ / \_\_ | | | | | | | | | |

| Sunday | Breakfast | | Lunch | | Dinner | | Bedtime | | Notes |
|---|---|---|---|---|---|---|---|---|---|
| | Before | After | Before | After | Before | After | Before | After | |
| \_\_ / \_\_ / \_\_ | | | | | | | | | |

| Week: _____ | | | | | | | | Weight: _____ |
|---|---|---|---|---|---|---|---|---|

| Monday | Breakfast | | Lunch | | Dinner | | Bedtime | | Notes |
|---|---|---|---|---|---|---|---|---|---|
| | Before | After | Before | After | Before | After | Before | After | |
| __ / __ / __ | | | | | | | | | |

| Tuesday | Breakfast | | Lunch | | Dinner | | Bedtime | | Notes |
|---|---|---|---|---|---|---|---|---|---|
| | Before | After | Before | After | Before | After | Before | After | |
| __ / __ / __ | | | | | | | | | |

| Wednesday | Breakfast | | Lunch | | Dinner | | Bedtime | | Notes |
|---|---|---|---|---|---|---|---|---|---|
| | Before | After | Before | After | Before | After | Before | After | |
| __ / __ / __ | | | | | | | | | |

| Thursday | Breakfast | | Lunch | | Dinner | | Bedtime | | Notes |
|---|---|---|---|---|---|---|---|---|---|
| | Before | After | Before | After | Before | After | Before | After | |
| __ / __ / __ | | | | | | | | | |

| Friday | Breakfast | | Lunch | | Dinner | | Bedtime | | Notes |
|---|---|---|---|---|---|---|---|---|---|
| | Before | After | Before | After | Before | After | Before | After | |
| __ / __ / __ | | | | | | | | | |

| Saturday | Breakfast | | Lunch | | Dinner | | Bedtime | | Notes |
|---|---|---|---|---|---|---|---|---|---|
| | Before | After | Before | After | Before | After | Before | After | |
| __ / __ / __ | | | | | | | | | |

| Sunday | Breakfast | | Lunch | | Dinner | | Bedtime | | Notes |
|---|---|---|---|---|---|---|---|---|---|
| | Before | After | Before | After | Before | After | Before | After | |
| __ / __ / __ | | | | | | | | | |

| Week: _____ | | | | | | | | | Weight: _____ |

| Monday | Breakfast | | Lunch | | Dinner | | Bedtime | | Notes |
|---|---|---|---|---|---|---|---|---|---|
| | Before | After | Before | After | Before | After | Before | After | |
| __/__/__ | | | | | | | | | |

| Tuesday | Breakfast | | Lunch | | Dinner | | Bedtime | | Notes |
|---|---|---|---|---|---|---|---|---|---|
| | Before | After | Before | After | Before | After | Before | After | |
| __/__/__ | | | | | | | | | |

| Wednesday | Breakfast | | Lunch | | Dinner | | Bedtime | | Notes |
|---|---|---|---|---|---|---|---|---|---|
| | Before | After | Before | After | Before | After | Before | After | |
| __/__/__ | | | | | | | | | |

| Thursday | Breakfast | | Lunch | | Dinner | | Bedtime | | Notes |
|---|---|---|---|---|---|---|---|---|---|
| | Before | After | Before | After | Before | After | Before | After | |
| __/__/__ | | | | | | | | | |

| Friday | Breakfast | | Lunch | | Dinner | | Bedtime | | Notes |
|---|---|---|---|---|---|---|---|---|---|
| | Before | After | Before | After | Before | After | Before | After | |
| __/__/__ | | | | | | | | | |

| Saturday | Breakfast | | Lunch | | Dinner | | Bedtime | | Notes |
|---|---|---|---|---|---|---|---|---|---|
| | Before | After | Before | After | Before | After | Before | After | |
| __/__/__ | | | | | | | | | |

| Sunday | Breakfast | | Lunch | | Dinner | | Bedtime | | Notes |
|---|---|---|---|---|---|---|---|---|---|
| | Before | After | Before | After | Before | After | Before | After | |
| __/__/__ | | | | | | | | | |

| Week: _____ | | | | | | | | | | Weight: _____ |

| Monday | Breakfast | | Lunch | | Dinner | | Bedtime | | Notes |
|--------|-----------|-------|-------|-------|--------|-------|---------|-------|-------|
| | Before | After | Before | After | Before | After | Before | After | |
| __/__/__ | | | | | | | | | |

| Tuesday | Breakfast | | Lunch | | Dinner | | Bedtime | | Notes |
|---------|-----------|-------|-------|-------|--------|-------|---------|-------|-------|
| | Before | After | Before | After | Before | After | Before | After | |
| __/__/__ | | | | | | | | | |

| Wednesday | Breakfast | | Lunch | | Dinner | | Bedtime | | Notes |
|-----------|-----------|-------|-------|-------|--------|-------|---------|-------|-------|
| | Before | After | Before | After | Before | After | Before | After | |
| __/__/__ | | | | | | | | | |

| Thursday | Breakfast | | Lunch | | Dinner | | Bedtime | | Notes |
|----------|-----------|-------|-------|-------|--------|-------|---------|-------|-------|
| | Before | After | Before | After | Before | After | Before | After | |
| __/__/__ | | | | | | | | | |

| Friday | Breakfast | | Lunch | | Dinner | | Bedtime | | Notes |
|--------|-----------|-------|-------|-------|--------|-------|---------|-------|-------|
| | Before | After | Before | After | Before | After | Before | After | |
| __/__/__ | | | | | | | | | |

| Saturday | Breakfast | | Lunch | | Dinner | | Bedtime | | Notes |
|----------|-----------|-------|-------|-------|--------|-------|---------|-------|-------|
| | Before | After | Before | After | Before | After | Before | After | |
| __/__/__ | | | | | | | | | |

| Sunday | Breakfast | | Lunch | | Dinner | | Bedtime | | Notes |
|--------|-----------|-------|-------|-------|--------|-------|---------|-------|-------|
| | Before | After | Before | After | Before | After | Before | After | |
| __/__/__ | | | | | | | | | |

| Week: _____ | | | | | | | | | Weight: _____ |

| Monday | Breakfast | | Lunch | | Dinner | | Bedtime | | Notes |
|---|---|---|---|---|---|---|---|---|---|
| | Before | After | Before | After | Before | After | Before | After | |
| __/__/__ | | | | | | | | | |

| Tuesday | Breakfast | | Lunch | | Dinner | | Bedtime | | Notes |
|---|---|---|---|---|---|---|---|---|---|
| | Before | After | Before | After | Before | After | Before | After | |
| __/__/__ | | | | | | | | | |

| Wednesday | Breakfast | | Lunch | | Dinner | | Bedtime | | Notes |
|---|---|---|---|---|---|---|---|---|---|
| | Before | After | Before | After | Before | After | Before | After | |
| __/__/__ | | | | | | | | | |

| Thursday | Breakfast | | Lunch | | Dinner | | Bedtime | | Notes |
|---|---|---|---|---|---|---|---|---|---|
| | Before | After | Before | After | Before | After | Before | After | |
| __/__/__ | | | | | | | | | |

| Friday | Breakfast | | Lunch | | Dinner | | Bedtime | | Notes |
|---|---|---|---|---|---|---|---|---|---|
| | Before | After | Before | After | Before | After | Before | After | |
| __/__/__ | | | | | | | | | |

| Saturday | Breakfast | | Lunch | | Dinner | | Bedtime | | Notes |
|---|---|---|---|---|---|---|---|---|---|
| | Before | After | Before | After | Before | After | Before | After | |
| __/__/__ | | | | | | | | | |

| Sunday | Breakfast | | Lunch | | Dinner | | Bedtime | | Notes |
|---|---|---|---|---|---|---|---|---|---|
| | Before | After | Before | After | Before | After | Before | After | |
| __/__/__ | | | | | | | | | |

| Monday | Breakfast | | Lunch | | Dinner | | Bedtime | | Notes |
|---|---|---|---|---|---|---|---|---|---|
| | Before | After | Before | After | Before | After | Before | After | |
| __/__/__ | | | | | | | | | |

| Tuesday | Breakfast | | Lunch | | Dinner | | Bedtime | | Notes |
|---|---|---|---|---|---|---|---|---|---|
| | Before | After | Before | After | Before | After | Before | After | |
| __/__/__ | | | | | | | | | |

| Wednesday | Breakfast | | Lunch | | Dinner | | Bedtime | | Notes |
|---|---|---|---|---|---|---|---|---|---|
| | Before | After | Before | After | Before | After | Before | After | |
| __/__/__ | | | | | | | | | |

| Thursday | Breakfast | | Lunch | | Dinner | | Bedtime | | Notes |
|---|---|---|---|---|---|---|---|---|---|
| | Before | After | Before | After | Before | After | Before | After | |
| __/__/__ | | | | | | | | | |

| Friday | Breakfast | | Lunch | | Dinner | | Bedtime | | Notes |
|---|---|---|---|---|---|---|---|---|---|
| | Before | After | Before | After | Before | After | Before | After | |
| __/__/__ | | | | | | | | | |

| Saturday | Breakfast | | Lunch | | Dinner | | Bedtime | | Notes |
|---|---|---|---|---|---|---|---|---|---|
| | Before | After | Before | After | Before | After | Before | After | |
| __/__/__ | | | | | | | | | |

| Sunday | Breakfast | | Lunch | | Dinner | | Bedtime | | Notes |
|---|---|---|---|---|---|---|---|---|---|
| | Before | After | Before | After | Before | After | Before | After | |
| __/__/__ | | | | | | | | | |

<table>
<tr><td>Week: _____</td><td></td><td></td><td></td><td>Weight: _____</td></tr>
</table>

| Monday | Breakfast | | Lunch | | Dinner | | Bedtime | | Notes |
|---|---|---|---|---|---|---|---|---|---|
| | Before | After | Before | After | Before | After | Before | After | |
| __/__/__ | | | | | | | | | |

| Tuesday | Breakfast | | Lunch | | Dinner | | Bedtime | | Notes |
|---|---|---|---|---|---|---|---|---|---|
| | Before | After | Before | After | Before | After | Before | After | |
| __/__/__ | | | | | | | | | |

| Wednesday | Breakfast | | Lunch | | Dinner | | Bedtime | | Notes |
|---|---|---|---|---|---|---|---|---|---|
| | Before | After | Before | After | Before | After | Before | After | |
| __/__/__ | | | | | | | | | |

| Thursday | Breakfast | | Lunch | | Dinner | | Bedtime | | Notes |
|---|---|---|---|---|---|---|---|---|---|
| | Before | After | Before | After | Before | After | Before | After | |
| __/__/__ | | | | | | | | | |

| Friday | Breakfast | | Lunch | | Dinner | | Bedtime | | Notes |
|---|---|---|---|---|---|---|---|---|---|
| | Before | After | Before | After | Before | After | Before | After | |
| __/__/__ | | | | | | | | | |

| Saturday | Breakfast | | Lunch | | Dinner | | Bedtime | | Notes |
|---|---|---|---|---|---|---|---|---|---|
| | Before | After | Before | After | Before | After | Before | After | |
| __/__/__ | | | | | | | | | |

| Sunday | Breakfast | | Lunch | | Dinner | | Bedtime | | Notes |
|---|---|---|---|---|---|---|---|---|---|
| | Before | After | Before | After | Before | After | Before | After | |
| __/__/__ | | | | | | | | | |

| Week: _____ | | | | | | | | | Weight: _____ |

| Monday | Breakfast | | Lunch | | Dinner | | Bedtime | | Notes |
|---|---|---|---|---|---|---|---|---|---|
| | Before | After | Before | After | Before | After | Before | After | |
| __ / __ / __ | | | | | | | | | |

| Tuesday | Breakfast | | Lunch | | Dinner | | Bedtime | | Notes |
|---|---|---|---|---|---|---|---|---|---|
| | Before | After | Before | After | Before | After | Before | After | |
| __ / __ / __ | | | | | | | | | |

| Wednesday | Breakfast | | Lunch | | Dinner | | Bedtime | | Notes |
|---|---|---|---|---|---|---|---|---|---|
| | Before | After | Before | After | Before | After | Before | After | |
| __ / __ / __ | | | | | | | | | |

| Thursday | Breakfast | | Lunch | | Dinner | | Bedtime | | Notes |
|---|---|---|---|---|---|---|---|---|---|
| | Before | After | Before | After | Before | After | Before | After | |
| __ / __ / __ | | | | | | | | | |

| Friday | Breakfast | | Lunch | | Dinner | | Bedtime | | Notes |
|---|---|---|---|---|---|---|---|---|---|
| | Before | After | Before | After | Before | After | Before | After | |
| __ / __ / __ | | | | | | | | | |

| Saturday | Breakfast | | Lunch | | Dinner | | Bedtime | | Notes |
|---|---|---|---|---|---|---|---|---|---|
| | Before | After | Before | After | Before | After | Before | After | |
| __ / __ / __ | | | | | | | | | |

| Sunday | Breakfast | | Lunch | | Dinner | | Bedtime | | Notes |
|---|---|---|---|---|---|---|---|---|---|
| | Before | After | Before | After | Before | After | Before | After | |
| __ / __ / __ | | | | | | | | | |

| Week: _____ | | | | | | | | | Weight: _____ |
|---|---|---|---|---|---|---|---|---|---|

| Monday | Breakfast | | Lunch | | Dinner | | Bedtime | | Notes |
|---|---|---|---|---|---|---|---|---|---|
| | Before | After | Before | After | Before | After | Before | After | |
| __ / __ / __ | | | | | | | | | |

| Tuesday | Breakfast | | Lunch | | Dinner | | Bedtime | | Notes |
|---|---|---|---|---|---|---|---|---|---|
| | Before | After | Before | After | Before | After | Before | After | |
| __ / __ / __ | | | | | | | | | |

| Wednesday | Breakfast | | Lunch | | Dinner | | Bedtime | | Notes |
|---|---|---|---|---|---|---|---|---|---|
| | Before | After | Before | After | Before | After | Before | After | |
| __ / __ / __ | | | | | | | | | |

| Thursday | Breakfast | | Lunch | | Dinner | | Bedtime | | Notes |
|---|---|---|---|---|---|---|---|---|---|
| | Before | After | Before | After | Before | After | Before | After | |
| __ / __ / __ | | | | | | | | | |

| Friday | Breakfast | | Lunch | | Dinner | | Bedtime | | Notes |
|---|---|---|---|---|---|---|---|---|---|
| | Before | After | Before | After | Before | After | Before | After | |
| __ / __ / __ | | | | | | | | | |

| Saturday | Breakfast | | Lunch | | Dinner | | Bedtime | | Notes |
|---|---|---|---|---|---|---|---|---|---|
| | Before | After | Before | After | Before | After | Before | After | |
| __ / __ / __ | | | | | | | | | |

| Sunday | Breakfast | | Lunch | | Dinner | | Bedtime | | Notes |
|---|---|---|---|---|---|---|---|---|---|
| | Before | After | Before | After | Before | After | Before | After | |
| __ / __ / __ | | | | | | | | | |

| Week: _____ | | | | | | | | | Weight: _____ |

| Monday | Breakfast | | Lunch | | Dinner | | Bedtime | | Notes |
|---|---|---|---|---|---|---|---|---|---|
| | Before | After | Before | After | Before | After | Before | After | |
| __/__/__ | | | | | | | | | |

| Tuesday | Breakfast | | Lunch | | Dinner | | Bedtime | | Notes |
|---|---|---|---|---|---|---|---|---|---|
| | Before | After | Before | After | Before | After | Before | After | |
| __/__/__ | | | | | | | | | |

| Wednesday | Breakfast | | Lunch | | Dinner | | Bedtime | | Notes |
|---|---|---|---|---|---|---|---|---|---|
| | Before | After | Before | After | Before | After | Before | After | |
| __/__/__ | | | | | | | | | |

| Thursday | Breakfast | | Lunch | | Dinner | | Bedtime | | Notes |
|---|---|---|---|---|---|---|---|---|---|
| | Before | After | Before | After | Before | After | Before | After | |
| __/__/__ | | | | | | | | | |

| Friday | Breakfast | | Lunch | | Dinner | | Bedtime | | Notes |
|---|---|---|---|---|---|---|---|---|---|
| | Before | After | Before | After | Before | After | Before | After | |
| __/__/__ | | | | | | | | | |

| Saturday | Breakfast | | Lunch | | Dinner | | Bedtime | | Notes |
|---|---|---|---|---|---|---|---|---|---|
| | Before | After | Before | After | Before | After | Before | After | |
| __/__/__ | | | | | | | | | |

| Sunday | Breakfast | | Lunch | | Dinner | | Bedtime | | Notes |
|---|---|---|---|---|---|---|---|---|---|
| | Before | After | Before | After | Before | After | Before | After | |
| __/__/__ | | | | | | | | | |

| Monday __/__/__ | Breakfast | | Lunch | | Dinner | | Bedtime | | Notes |
|---|---|---|---|---|---|---|---|---|---|
| | Before | After | Before | After | Before | After | Before | After | |
| | | | | | | | | | |

| Tuesday __/__/__ | Breakfast | | Lunch | | Dinner | | Bedtime | | Notes |
|---|---|---|---|---|---|---|---|---|---|
| | Before | After | Before | After | Before | After | Before | After | |
| | | | | | | | | | |

| Wednesday __/__/__ | Breakfast | | Lunch | | Dinner | | Bedtime | | Notes |
|---|---|---|---|---|---|---|---|---|---|
| | Before | After | Before | After | Before | After | Before | After | |
| | | | | | | | | | |

| Thursday __/__/__ | Breakfast | | Lunch | | Dinner | | Bedtime | | Notes |
|---|---|---|---|---|---|---|---|---|---|
| | Before | After | Before | After | Before | After | Before | After | |
| | | | | | | | | | |

| Friday __/__/__ | Breakfast | | Lunch | | Dinner | | Bedtime | | Notes |
|---|---|---|---|---|---|---|---|---|---|
| | Before | After | Before | After | Before | After | Before | After | |
| | | | | | | | | | |

| Saturday __/__/__ | Breakfast | | Lunch | | Dinner | | Bedtime | | Notes |
|---|---|---|---|---|---|---|---|---|---|
| | Before | After | Before | After | Before | After | Before | After | |
| | | | | | | | | | |

| Sunday __/__/__ | Breakfast | | Lunch | | Dinner | | Bedtime | | Notes |
|---|---|---|---|---|---|---|---|---|---|
| | Before | After | Before | After | Before | After | Before | After | |
| | | | | | | | | | |

| Monday __ / __ / __ | Breakfast | | Lunch | | Dinner | | Bedtime | | Notes |
|---|---|---|---|---|---|---|---|---|---|
| | Before | After | Before | After | Before | After | Before | After | |
| | | | | | | | | | |

| Tuesday __ / __ / __ | Breakfast | | Lunch | | Dinner | | Bedtime | | Notes |
|---|---|---|---|---|---|---|---|---|---|
| | Before | After | Before | After | Before | After | Before | After | |
| | | | | | | | | | |

| Wednesday __ / __ / __ | Breakfast | | Lunch | | Dinner | | Bedtime | | Notes |
|---|---|---|---|---|---|---|---|---|---|
| | Before | After | Before | After | Before | After | Before | After | |
| | | | | | | | | | |

| Thursday __ / __ / __ | Breakfast | | Lunch | | Dinner | | Bedtime | | Notes |
|---|---|---|---|---|---|---|---|---|---|
| | Before | After | Before | After | Before | After | Before | After | |
| | | | | | | | | | |

| Friday __ / __ / __ | Breakfast | | Lunch | | Dinner | | Bedtime | | Notes |
|---|---|---|---|---|---|---|---|---|---|
| | Before | After | Before | After | Before | After | Before | After | |
| | | | | | | | | | |

| Saturday __ / __ / __ | Breakfast | | Lunch | | Dinner | | Bedtime | | Notes |
|---|---|---|---|---|---|---|---|---|---|
| | Before | After | Before | After | Before | After | Before | After | |
| | | | | | | | | | |

| Sunday __ / __ / __ | Breakfast | | Lunch | | Dinner | | Bedtime | | Notes |
|---|---|---|---|---|---|---|---|---|---|
| | Before | After | Before | After | Before | After | Before | After | |
| | | | | | | | | | |

| Week: _____ | | | | | | | | | Weight: _____ |

| Monday | Breakfast | | Lunch | | Dinner | | Bedtime | | Notes |
|---|---|---|---|---|---|---|---|---|---|
| | Before | After | Before | After | Before | After | Before | After | |
| __/__/__ | | | | | | | | | |

| Tuesday | Breakfast | | Lunch | | Dinner | | Bedtime | | Notes |
|---|---|---|---|---|---|---|---|---|---|
| | Before | After | Before | After | Before | After | Before | After | |
| __/__/__ | | | | | | | | | |

| Wednesday | Breakfast | | Lunch | | Dinner | | Bedtime | | Notes |
|---|---|---|---|---|---|---|---|---|---|
| | Before | After | Before | After | Before | After | Before | After | |
| __/__/__ | | | | | | | | | |

| Thursday | Breakfast | | Lunch | | Dinner | | Bedtime | | Notes |
|---|---|---|---|---|---|---|---|---|---|
| | Before | After | Before | After | Before | After | Before | After | |
| __/__/__ | | | | | | | | | |

| Friday | Breakfast | | Lunch | | Dinner | | Bedtime | | Notes |
|---|---|---|---|---|---|---|---|---|---|
| | Before | After | Before | After | Before | After | Before | After | |
| __/__/__ | | | | | | | | | |

| Saturday | Breakfast | | Lunch | | Dinner | | Bedtime | | Notes |
|---|---|---|---|---|---|---|---|---|---|
| | Before | After | Before | After | Before | After | Before | After | |
| __/__/__ | | | | | | | | | |

| Sunday | Breakfast | | Lunch | | Dinner | | Bedtime | | Notes |
|---|---|---|---|---|---|---|---|---|---|
| | Before | After | Before | After | Before | After | Before | After | |
| __/__/__ | | | | | | | | | |

| Week: _____ | | | | | | | | | Weight: _____ |
|---|---|---|---|---|---|---|---|---|---|

| Monday | Breakfast | | Lunch | | Dinner | | Bedtime | | Notes |
|---|---|---|---|---|---|---|---|---|---|
| | Before | After | Before | After | Before | After | Before | After | |
| __ / __ / __ | | | | | | | | | |

| Tuesday | Breakfast | | Lunch | | Dinner | | Bedtime | | Notes |
|---|---|---|---|---|---|---|---|---|---|
| | Before | After | Before | After | Before | After | Before | After | |
| __ / __ / __ | | | | | | | | | |

| Wednesday | Breakfast | | Lunch | | Dinner | | Bedtime | | Notes |
|---|---|---|---|---|---|---|---|---|---|
| | Before | After | Before | After | Before | After | Before | After | |
| __ / __ / __ | | | | | | | | | |

| Thursday | Breakfast | | Lunch | | Dinner | | Bedtime | | Notes |
|---|---|---|---|---|---|---|---|---|---|
| | Before | After | Before | After | Before | After | Before | After | |
| __ / __ / __ | | | | | | | | | |

| Friday | Breakfast | | Lunch | | Dinner | | Bedtime | | Notes |
|---|---|---|---|---|---|---|---|---|---|
| | Before | After | Before | After | Before | After | Before | After | |
| __ / __ / __ | | | | | | | | | |

| Saturday | Breakfast | | Lunch | | Dinner | | Bedtime | | Notes |
|---|---|---|---|---|---|---|---|---|---|
| | Before | After | Before | After | Before | After | Before | After | |
| __ / __ / __ | | | | | | | | | |

| Sunday | Breakfast | | Lunch | | Dinner | | Bedtime | | Notes |
|---|---|---|---|---|---|---|---|---|---|
| | Before | After | Before | After | Before | After | Before | After | |
| __ / __ / __ | | | | | | | | | |

| Monday | Breakfast | | Lunch | | Dinner | | Bedtime | | Notes |
|---|---|---|---|---|---|---|---|---|---|
| | Before | After | Before | After | Before | After | Before | After | |
| __/__/__ | | | | | | | | | |

| Tuesday | Breakfast | | Lunch | | Dinner | | Bedtime | | Notes |
|---|---|---|---|---|---|---|---|---|---|
| | Before | After | Before | After | Before | After | Before | After | |
| __/__/__ | | | | | | | | | |

| Wednesday | Breakfast | | Lunch | | Dinner | | Bedtime | | Notes |
|---|---|---|---|---|---|---|---|---|---|
| | Before | After | Before | After | Before | After | Before | After | |
| __/__/__ | | | | | | | | | |

| Thursday | Breakfast | | Lunch | | Dinner | | Bedtime | | Notes |
|---|---|---|---|---|---|---|---|---|---|
| | Before | After | Before | After | Before | After | Before | After | |
| __/__/__ | | | | | | | | | |

| Friday | Breakfast | | Lunch | | Dinner | | Bedtime | | Notes |
|---|---|---|---|---|---|---|---|---|---|
| | Before | After | Before | After | Before | After | Before | After | |
| __/__/__ | | | | | | | | | |

| Saturday | Breakfast | | Lunch | | Dinner | | Bedtime | | Notes |
|---|---|---|---|---|---|---|---|---|---|
| | Before | After | Before | After | Before | After | Before | After | |
| __/__/__ | | | | | | | | | |

| Sunday | Breakfast | | Lunch | | Dinner | | Bedtime | | Notes |
|---|---|---|---|---|---|---|---|---|---|
| | Before | After | Before | After | Before | After | Before | After | |
| __/__/__ | | | | | | | | | |

| Week: _____ | | | | | | | | | Weight: _____ |

| Monday | Breakfast | | Lunch | | Dinner | | Bedtime | | Notes |
|---|---|---|---|---|---|---|---|---|---|
| | Before | After | Before | After | Before | After | Before | After | |
| __ / __ / __ | | | | | | | | | |

| Tuesday | Breakfast | | Lunch | | Dinner | | Bedtime | | Notes |
|---|---|---|---|---|---|---|---|---|---|
| | Before | After | Before | After | Before | After | Before | After | |
| __ / __ / __ | | | | | | | | | |

| Wednesday | Breakfast | | Lunch | | Dinner | | Bedtime | | Notes |
|---|---|---|---|---|---|---|---|---|---|
| | Before | After | Before | After | Before | After | Before | After | |
| __ / __ / __ | | | | | | | | | |

| Thursday | Breakfast | | Lunch | | Dinner | | Bedtime | | Notes |
|---|---|---|---|---|---|---|---|---|---|
| | Before | After | Before | After | Before | After | Before | After | |
| __ / __ / __ | | | | | | | | | |

| Friday | Breakfast | | Lunch | | Dinner | | Bedtime | | Notes |
|---|---|---|---|---|---|---|---|---|---|
| | Before | After | Before | After | Before | After | Before | After | |
| __ / __ / __ | | | | | | | | | |

| Saturday | Breakfast | | Lunch | | Dinner | | Bedtime | | Notes |
|---|---|---|---|---|---|---|---|---|---|
| | Before | After | Before | After | Before | After | Before | After | |
| __ / __ / __ | | | | | | | | | |

| Sunday | Breakfast | | Lunch | | Dinner | | Bedtime | | Notes |
|---|---|---|---|---|---|---|---|---|---|
| | Before | After | Before | After | Before | After | Before | After | |
| __ / __ / __ | | | | | | | | | |

<table>
<tr><td>Week: _____</td><td colspan="8"></td><td>Weight: _____</td></tr>
</table>

| Monday | Breakfast | | Lunch | | Dinner | | Bedtime | | Notes |
|---|---|---|---|---|---|---|---|---|---|
| | Before | After | Before | After | Before | After | Before | After | |
| __/__/__ | | | | | | | | | |

| Tuesday | Breakfast | | Lunch | | Dinner | | Bedtime | | Notes |
|---|---|---|---|---|---|---|---|---|---|
| | Before | After | Before | After | Before | After | Before | After | |
| __/__/__ | | | | | | | | | |

| Wednesday | Breakfast | | Lunch | | Dinner | | Bedtime | | Notes |
|---|---|---|---|---|---|---|---|---|---|
| | Before | After | Before | After | Before | After | Before | After | |
| __/__/__ | | | | | | | | | |

| Thursday | Breakfast | | Lunch | | Dinner | | Bedtime | | Notes |
|---|---|---|---|---|---|---|---|---|---|
| | Before | After | Before | After | Before | After | Before | After | |
| __/__/__ | | | | | | | | | |

| Friday | Breakfast | | Lunch | | Dinner | | Bedtime | | Notes |
|---|---|---|---|---|---|---|---|---|---|
| | Before | After | Before | After | Before | After | Before | After | |
| __/__/__ | | | | | | | | | |

| Saturday | Breakfast | | Lunch | | Dinner | | Bedtime | | Notes |
|---|---|---|---|---|---|---|---|---|---|
| | Before | After | Before | After | Before | After | Before | After | |
| __/__/__ | | | | | | | | | |

| Sunday | Breakfast | | Lunch | | Dinner | | Bedtime | | Notes |
|---|---|---|---|---|---|---|---|---|---|
| | Before | After | Before | After | Before | After | Before | After | |
| __/__/__ | | | | | | | | | |

| Week: _____ | | | | | | | | | Weight: _____ |
|---|---|---|---|---|---|---|---|---|---|

| Monday | Breakfast | | Lunch | | Dinner | | Bedtime | | Notes |
|---|---|---|---|---|---|---|---|---|---|
| | Before | After | Before | After | Before | After | Before | After | |
| __ / __ / __ | | | | | | | | | |

| Tuesday | Breakfast | | Lunch | | Dinner | | Bedtime | | Notes |
|---|---|---|---|---|---|---|---|---|---|
| | Before | After | Before | After | Before | After | Before | After | |
| __ / __ / __ | | | | | | | | | |

| Wednesday | Breakfast | | Lunch | | Dinner | | Bedtime | | Notes |
|---|---|---|---|---|---|---|---|---|---|
| | Before | After | Before | After | Before | After | Before | After | |
| __ / __ / __ | | | | | | | | | |

| Thursday | Breakfast | | Lunch | | Dinner | | Bedtime | | Notes |
|---|---|---|---|---|---|---|---|---|---|
| | Before | After | Before | After | Before | After | Before | After | |
| __ / __ / __ | | | | | | | | | |

| Friday | Breakfast | | Lunch | | Dinner | | Bedtime | | Notes |
|---|---|---|---|---|---|---|---|---|---|
| | Before | After | Before | After | Before | After | Before | After | |
| __ / __ / __ | | | | | | | | | |

| Saturday | Breakfast | | Lunch | | Dinner | | Bedtime | | Notes |
|---|---|---|---|---|---|---|---|---|---|
| | Before | After | Before | After | Before | After | Before | After | |
| __ / __ / __ | | | | | | | | | |

| Sunday | Breakfast | | Lunch | | Dinner | | Bedtime | | Notes |
|---|---|---|---|---|---|---|---|---|---|
| | Before | After | Before | After | Before | After | Before | After | |
| __ / __ / __ | | | | | | | | | |

| Monday | Breakfast | | Lunch | | Dinner | | Bedtime | | Notes |
|---|---|---|---|---|---|---|---|---|---|
| | Before | After | Before | After | Before | After | Before | After | |
| __ / __ / __ | | | | | | | | | |

| Tuesday | Breakfast | | Lunch | | Dinner | | Bedtime | | Notes |
|---|---|---|---|---|---|---|---|---|---|
| | Before | After | Before | After | Before | After | Before | After | |
| __ / __ / __ | | | | | | | | | |

| Wednesday | Breakfast | | Lunch | | Dinner | | Bedtime | | Notes |
|---|---|---|---|---|---|---|---|---|---|
| | Before | After | Before | After | Before | After | Before | After | |
| __ / __ / __ | | | | | | | | | |

| Thursday | Breakfast | | Lunch | | Dinner | | Bedtime | | Notes |
|---|---|---|---|---|---|---|---|---|---|
| | Before | After | Before | After | Before | After | Before | After | |
| __ / __ / __ | | | | | | | | | |

| Friday | Breakfast | | Lunch | | Dinner | | Bedtime | | Notes |
|---|---|---|---|---|---|---|---|---|---|
| | Before | After | Before | After | Before | After | Before | After | |
| __ / __ / __ | | | | | | | | | |

| Saturday | Breakfast | | Lunch | | Dinner | | Bedtime | | Notes |
|---|---|---|---|---|---|---|---|---|---|
| | Before | After | Before | After | Before | After | Before | After | |
| __ / __ / __ | | | | | | | | | |

| Sunday | Breakfast | | Lunch | | Dinner | | Bedtime | | Notes |
|---|---|---|---|---|---|---|---|---|---|
| | Before | After | Before | After | Before | After | Before | After | |
| __ / __ / __ | | | | | | | | | |

| Week: _____ | | | | | | | | | Weight: _____ |
|---|---|---|---|---|---|---|---|---|---|

| Monday | Breakfast | | Lunch | | Dinner | | Bedtime | | Notes |
|---|---|---|---|---|---|---|---|---|---|
| | Before | After | Before | After | Before | After | Before | After | |
| __ / __ / __ | | | | | | | | | |

| Tuesday | Breakfast | | Lunch | | Dinner | | Bedtime | | Notes |
|---|---|---|---|---|---|---|---|---|---|
| | Before | After | Before | After | Before | After | Before | After | |
| __ / __ / __ | | | | | | | | | |

| Wednesday | Breakfast | | Lunch | | Dinner | | Bedtime | | Notes |
|---|---|---|---|---|---|---|---|---|---|
| | Before | After | Before | After | Before | After | Before | After | |
| __ / __ / __ | | | | | | | | | |

| Thursday | Breakfast | | Lunch | | Dinner | | Bedtime | | Notes |
|---|---|---|---|---|---|---|---|---|---|
| | Before | After | Before | After | Before | After | Before | After | |
| __ / __ / __ | | | | | | | | | |

| Friday | Breakfast | | Lunch | | Dinner | | Bedtime | | Notes |
|---|---|---|---|---|---|---|---|---|---|
| | Before | After | Before | After | Before | After | Before | After | |
| __ / __ / __ | | | | | | | | | |

| Saturday | Breakfast | | Lunch | | Dinner | | Bedtime | | Notes |
|---|---|---|---|---|---|---|---|---|---|
| | Before | After | Before | After | Before | After | Before | After | |
| __ / __ / __ | | | | | | | | | |

| Sunday | Breakfast | | Lunch | | Dinner | | Bedtime | | Notes |
|---|---|---|---|---|---|---|---|---|---|
| | Before | After | Before | After | Before | After | Before | After | |
| __ / __ / __ | | | | | | | | | |

| Week: _____ | | | | | | | | | Weight: _____ | |
|---|---|---|---|---|---|---|---|---|---|---|

| Monday | Breakfast | | Lunch | | Dinner | | Bedtime | | Notes |
|---|---|---|---|---|---|---|---|---|---|
| | Before | After | Before | After | Before | After | Before | After | |
| __ / __ / __ | | | | | | | | | |

| Tuesday | Breakfast | | Lunch | | Dinner | | Bedtime | | Notes |
|---|---|---|---|---|---|---|---|---|---|
| | Before | After | Before | After | Before | After | Before | After | |
| __ / __ / __ | | | | | | | | | |

| Wednesday | Breakfast | | Lunch | | Dinner | | Bedtime | | Notes |
|---|---|---|---|---|---|---|---|---|---|
| | Before | After | Before | After | Before | After | Before | After | |
| __ / __ / __ | | | | | | | | | |

| Thursday | Breakfast | | Lunch | | Dinner | | Bedtime | | Notes |
|---|---|---|---|---|---|---|---|---|---|
| | Before | After | Before | After | Before | After | Before | After | |
| __ / __ / __ | | | | | | | | | |

| Friday | Breakfast | | Lunch | | Dinner | | Bedtime | | Notes |
|---|---|---|---|---|---|---|---|---|---|
| | Before | After | Before | After | Before | After | Before | After | |
| __ / __ / __ | | | | | | | | | |

| Saturday | Breakfast | | Lunch | | Dinner | | Bedtime | | Notes |
|---|---|---|---|---|---|---|---|---|---|
| | Before | After | Before | After | Before | After | Before | After | |
| __ / __ / __ | | | | | | | | | |

| Sunday | Breakfast | | Lunch | | Dinner | | Bedtime | | Notes |
|---|---|---|---|---|---|---|---|---|---|
| | Before | After | Before | After | Before | After | Before | After | |
| __ / __ / __ | | | | | | | | | |

| Week: _____ | | | | | | | | | Weight: _____ |
|---|---|---|---|---|---|---|---|---|---|

| Monday | Breakfast | | Lunch | | Dinner | | Bedtime | | Notes |
|---|---|---|---|---|---|---|---|---|---|
| | Before | After | Before | After | Before | After | Before | After | |
| __ / __ / __ | | | | | | | | | |

| Tuesday | Breakfast | | Lunch | | Dinner | | Bedtime | | Notes |
|---|---|---|---|---|---|---|---|---|---|
| | Before | After | Before | After | Before | After | Before | After | |
| __ / __ / __ | | | | | | | | | |

| Wednesday | Breakfast | | Lunch | | Dinner | | Bedtime | | Notes |
|---|---|---|---|---|---|---|---|---|---|
| | Before | After | Before | After | Before | After | Before | After | |
| __ / __ / __ | | | | | | | | | |

| Thursday | Breakfast | | Lunch | | Dinner | | Bedtime | | Notes |
|---|---|---|---|---|---|---|---|---|---|
| | Before | After | Before | After | Before | After | Before | After | |
| __ / __ / __ | | | | | | | | | |

| Friday | Breakfast | | Lunch | | Dinner | | Bedtime | | Notes |
|---|---|---|---|---|---|---|---|---|---|
| | Before | After | Before | After | Before | After | Before | After | |
| __ / __ / __ | | | | | | | | | |

| Saturday | Breakfast | | Lunch | | Dinner | | Bedtime | | Notes |
|---|---|---|---|---|---|---|---|---|---|
| | Before | After | Before | After | Before | After | Before | After | |
| __ / __ / __ | | | | | | | | | |

| Sunday | Breakfast | | Lunch | | Dinner | | Bedtime | | Notes |
|---|---|---|---|---|---|---|---|---|---|
| | Before | After | Before | After | Before | After | Before | After | |
| __ / __ / __ | | | | | | | | | |

| Week: _____ | | | | | | | | | Weight: _____ |
|---|---|---|---|---|---|---|---|---|---|

| Monday | Breakfast | | Lunch | | Dinner | | Bedtime | | Notes |
|---|---|---|---|---|---|---|---|---|---|
| | Before | After | Before | After | Before | After | Before | After | |
| __ / __ / __ | | | | | | | | | |

| Tuesday | Breakfast | | Lunch | | Dinner | | Bedtime | | Notes |
|---|---|---|---|---|---|---|---|---|---|
| | Before | After | Before | After | Before | After | Before | After | |
| __ / __ / __ | | | | | | | | | |

| Wednesday | Breakfast | | Lunch | | Dinner | | Bedtime | | Notes |
|---|---|---|---|---|---|---|---|---|---|
| | Before | After | Before | After | Before | After | Before | After | |
| __ / __ / __ | | | | | | | | | |

| Thursday | Breakfast | | Lunch | | Dinner | | Bedtime | | Notes |
|---|---|---|---|---|---|---|---|---|---|
| | Before | After | Before | After | Before | After | Before | After | |
| __ / __ / __ | | | | | | | | | |

| Friday | Breakfast | | Lunch | | Dinner | | Bedtime | | Notes |
|---|---|---|---|---|---|---|---|---|---|
| | Before | After | Before | After | Before | After | Before | After | |
| __ / __ / __ | | | | | | | | | |

| Saturday | Breakfast | | Lunch | | Dinner | | Bedtime | | Notes |
|---|---|---|---|---|---|---|---|---|---|
| | Before | After | Before | After | Before | After | Before | After | |
| __ / __ / __ | | | | | | | | | |

| Sunday | Breakfast | | Lunch | | Dinner | | Bedtime | | Notes |
|---|---|---|---|---|---|---|---|---|---|
| | Before | After | Before | After | Before | After | Before | After | |
| __ / __ / __ | | | | | | | | | |

| Week: _____ | | | | | | | | | Weight: _____ |

| Monday | Breakfast | | Lunch | | Dinner | | Bedtime | | Notes |
|---|---|---|---|---|---|---|---|---|---|
| | Before | After | Before | After | Before | After | Before | After | |
| __ / __ / __ | | | | | | | | | |

| Tuesday | Breakfast | | Lunch | | Dinner | | Bedtime | | Notes |
|---|---|---|---|---|---|---|---|---|---|
| | Before | After | Before | After | Before | After | Before | After | |
| __ / __ / __ | | | | | | | | | |

| Wednesday | Breakfast | | Lunch | | Dinner | | Bedtime | | Notes |
|---|---|---|---|---|---|---|---|---|---|
| | Before | After | Before | After | Before | After | Before | After | |
| __ / __ / __ | | | | | | | | | |

| Thursday | Breakfast | | Lunch | | Dinner | | Bedtime | | Notes |
|---|---|---|---|---|---|---|---|---|---|
| | Before | After | Before | After | Before | After | Before | After | |
| __ / __ / __ | | | | | | | | | |

| Friday | Breakfast | | Lunch | | Dinner | | Bedtime | | Notes |
|---|---|---|---|---|---|---|---|---|---|
| | Before | After | Before | After | Before | After | Before | After | |
| __ / __ / __ | | | | | | | | | |

| Saturday | Breakfast | | Lunch | | Dinner | | Bedtime | | Notes |
|---|---|---|---|---|---|---|---|---|---|
| | Before | After | Before | After | Before | After | Before | After | |
| __ / __ / __ | | | | | | | | | |

| Sunday | Breakfast | | Lunch | | Dinner | | Bedtime | | Notes |
|---|---|---|---|---|---|---|---|---|---|
| | Before | After | Before | After | Before | After | Before | After | |
| __ / __ / __ | | | | | | | | | |

| Week: _____ | | | | | | | | | Weight: _____ |

| Monday | Breakfast | | Lunch | | Dinner | | Bedtime | | Notes |
|---|---|---|---|---|---|---|---|---|---|
| | Before | After | Before | After | Before | After | Before | After | |
| __ / __ / __ | | | | | | | | | |

| Tuesday | Breakfast | | Lunch | | Dinner | | Bedtime | | Notes |
|---|---|---|---|---|---|---|---|---|---|
| | Before | After | Before | After | Before | After | Before | After | |
| __ / __ / __ | | | | | | | | | |

| Wednesday | Breakfast | | Lunch | | Dinner | | Bedtime | | Notes |
|---|---|---|---|---|---|---|---|---|---|
| | Before | After | Before | After | Before | After | Before | After | |
| __ / __ / __ | | | | | | | | | |

| Thursday | Breakfast | | Lunch | | Dinner | | Bedtime | | Notes |
|---|---|---|---|---|---|---|---|---|---|
| | Before | After | Before | After | Before | After | Before | After | |
| __ / __ / __ | | | | | | | | | |

| Friday | Breakfast | | Lunch | | Dinner | | Bedtime | | Notes |
|---|---|---|---|---|---|---|---|---|---|
| | Before | After | Before | After | Before | After | Before | After | |
| __ / __ / __ | | | | | | | | | |

| Saturday | Breakfast | | Lunch | | Dinner | | Bedtime | | Notes |
|---|---|---|---|---|---|---|---|---|---|
| | Before | After | Before | After | Before | After | Before | After | |
| __ / __ / __ | | | | | | | | | |

| Sunday | Breakfast | | Lunch | | Dinner | | Bedtime | | Notes |
|---|---|---|---|---|---|---|---|---|---|
| | Before | After | Before | After | Before | After | Before | After | |
| __ / __ / __ | | | | | | | | | |

| Week: _____ | | | | | | | | | Weight: _____ |

| Monday | Breakfast | | Lunch | | Dinner | | Bedtime | | Notes |
|---|---|---|---|---|---|---|---|---|---|
| | Before | After | Before | After | Before | After | Before | After | |
| __ / __ / __ | | | | | | | | | |

| Tuesday | Breakfast | | Lunch | | Dinner | | Bedtime | | Notes |
|---|---|---|---|---|---|---|---|---|---|
| | Before | After | Before | After | Before | After | Before | After | |
| __ / __ / __ | | | | | | | | | |

| Wednesday | Breakfast | | Lunch | | Dinner | | Bedtime | | Notes |
|---|---|---|---|---|---|---|---|---|---|
| | Before | After | Before | After | Before | After | Before | After | |
| __ / __ / __ | | | | | | | | | |

| Thursday | Breakfast | | Lunch | | Dinner | | Bedtime | | Notes |
|---|---|---|---|---|---|---|---|---|---|
| | Before | After | Before | After | Before | After | Before | After | |
| __ / __ / __ | | | | | | | | | |

| Friday | Breakfast | | Lunch | | Dinner | | Bedtime | | Notes |
|---|---|---|---|---|---|---|---|---|---|
| | Before | After | Before | After | Before | After | Before | After | |
| __ / __ / __ | | | | | | | | | |

| Saturday | Breakfast | | Lunch | | Dinner | | Bedtime | | Notes |
|---|---|---|---|---|---|---|---|---|---|
| | Before | After | Before | After | Before | After | Before | After | |
| __ / __ / __ | | | | | | | | | |

| Sunday | Breakfast | | Lunch | | Dinner | | Bedtime | | Notes |
|---|---|---|---|---|---|---|---|---|---|
| | Before | After | Before | After | Before | After | Before | After | |
| __ / __ / __ | | | | | | | | | |

| Week: _____ | | | | | | | | | Weight: _____ |
|---|---|---|---|---|---|---|---|---|---|

| Monday | Breakfast | | Lunch | | Dinner | | Bedtime | | Notes |
|---|---|---|---|---|---|---|---|---|---|
| | Before | After | Before | After | Before | After | Before | After | |
| __/__/__ | | | | | | | | | |

| Tuesday | Breakfast | | Lunch | | Dinner | | Bedtime | | Notes |
|---|---|---|---|---|---|---|---|---|---|
| | Before | After | Before | After | Before | After | Before | After | |
| __/__/__ | | | | | | | | | |

| Wednesday | Breakfast | | Lunch | | Dinner | | Bedtime | | Notes |
|---|---|---|---|---|---|---|---|---|---|
| | Before | After | Before | After | Before | After | Before | After | |
| __/__/__ | | | | | | | | | |

| Thursday | Breakfast | | Lunch | | Dinner | | Bedtime | | Notes |
|---|---|---|---|---|---|---|---|---|---|
| | Before | After | Before | After | Before | After | Before | After | |
| __/__/__ | | | | | | | | | |

| Friday | Breakfast | | Lunch | | Dinner | | Bedtime | | Notes |
|---|---|---|---|---|---|---|---|---|---|
| | Before | After | Before | After | Before | After | Before | After | |
| __/__/__ | | | | | | | | | |

| Saturday | Breakfast | | Lunch | | Dinner | | Bedtime | | Notes |
|---|---|---|---|---|---|---|---|---|---|
| | Before | After | Before | After | Before | After | Before | After | |
| __/__/__ | | | | | | | | | |

| Sunday | Breakfast | | Lunch | | Dinner | | Bedtime | | Notes |
|---|---|---|---|---|---|---|---|---|---|
| | Before | After | Before | After | Before | After | Before | After | |
| __/__/__ | | | | | | | | | |

| Week: _____ | | | | | | | | | Weight: _____ |
|---|---|---|---|---|---|---|---|---|---|

| Monday | Breakfast | | Lunch | | Dinner | | Bedtime | | Notes |
|---|---|---|---|---|---|---|---|---|---|
| | Before | After | Before | After | Before | After | Before | After | |
| __ / __ / __ | | | | | | | | | |

| Tuesday | Breakfast | | Lunch | | Dinner | | Bedtime | | Notes |
|---|---|---|---|---|---|---|---|---|---|
| | Before | After | Before | After | Before | After | Before | After | |
| __ / __ / __ | | | | | | | | | |

| Wednesday | Breakfast | | Lunch | | Dinner | | Bedtime | | Notes |
|---|---|---|---|---|---|---|---|---|---|
| | Before | After | Before | After | Before | After | Before | After | |
| __ / __ / __ | | | | | | | | | |

| Thursday | Breakfast | | Lunch | | Dinner | | Bedtime | | Notes |
|---|---|---|---|---|---|---|---|---|---|
| | Before | After | Before | After | Before | After | Before | After | |
| __ / __ / __ | | | | | | | | | |

| Friday | Breakfast | | Lunch | | Dinner | | Bedtime | | Notes |
|---|---|---|---|---|---|---|---|---|---|
| | Before | After | Before | After | Before | After | Before | After | |
| __ / __ / __ | | | | | | | | | |

| Saturday | Breakfast | | Lunch | | Dinner | | Bedtime | | Notes |
|---|---|---|---|---|---|---|---|---|---|
| | Before | After | Before | After | Before | After | Before | After | |
| __ / __ / __ | | | | | | | | | |

| Sunday | Breakfast | | Lunch | | Dinner | | Bedtime | | Notes |
|---|---|---|---|---|---|---|---|---|---|
| | Before | After | Before | After | Before | After | Before | After | |
| __ / __ / __ | | | | | | | | | |

| Week: _____ | | | | | | | | | Weight: _____ |
|---|---|---|---|---|---|---|---|---|---|

| Monday | Breakfast | | Lunch | | Dinner | | Bedtime | | Notes |
|---|---|---|---|---|---|---|---|---|---|
| | Before | After | Before | After | Before | After | Before | After | |
| \_\_ / \_\_ / \_\_ | | | | | | | | | |

| Tuesday | Breakfast | | Lunch | | Dinner | | Bedtime | | Notes |
|---|---|---|---|---|---|---|---|---|---|
| | Before | After | Before | After | Before | After | Before | After | |
| \_\_ / \_\_ / \_\_ | | | | | | | | | |

| Wednesday | Breakfast | | Lunch | | Dinner | | Bedtime | | Notes |
|---|---|---|---|---|---|---|---|---|---|
| | Before | After | Before | After | Before | After | Before | After | |
| \_\_ / \_\_ / \_\_ | | | | | | | | | |

| Thursday | Breakfast | | Lunch | | Dinner | | Bedtime | | Notes |
|---|---|---|---|---|---|---|---|---|---|
| | Before | After | Before | After | Before | After | Before | After | |
| \_\_ / \_\_ / \_\_ | | | | | | | | | |

| Friday | Breakfast | | Lunch | | Dinner | | Bedtime | | Notes |
|---|---|---|---|---|---|---|---|---|---|
| | Before | After | Before | After | Before | After | Before | After | |
| \_\_ / \_\_ / \_\_ | | | | | | | | | |

| Saturday | Breakfast | | Lunch | | Dinner | | Bedtime | | Notes |
|---|---|---|---|---|---|---|---|---|---|
| | Before | After | Before | After | Before | After | Before | After | |
| \_\_ / \_\_ / \_\_ | | | | | | | | | |

| Sunday | Breakfast | | Lunch | | Dinner | | Bedtime | | Notes |
|---|---|---|---|---|---|---|---|---|---|
| | Before | After | Before | After | Before | After | Before | After | |
| \_\_ / \_\_ / \_\_ | | | | | | | | | |

| Week: _____ | | | | | | | | | Weight: _____ |
|---|---|---|---|---|---|---|---|---|---|

| Monday | Breakfast | | Lunch | | Dinner | | Bedtime | | Notes |
|---|---|---|---|---|---|---|---|---|---|
| | Before | After | Before | After | Before | After | Before | After | |
| __ / __ / __ | | | | | | | | | |

| Tuesday | Breakfast | | Lunch | | Dinner | | Bedtime | | Notes |
|---|---|---|---|---|---|---|---|---|---|
| | Before | After | Before | After | Before | After | Before | After | |
| __ / __ / __ | | | | | | | | | |

| Wednesday | Breakfast | | Lunch | | Dinner | | Bedtime | | Notes |
|---|---|---|---|---|---|---|---|---|---|
| | Before | After | Before | After | Before | After | Before | After | |
| __ / __ / __ | | | | | | | | | |

| Thursday | Breakfast | | Lunch | | Dinner | | Bedtime | | Notes |
|---|---|---|---|---|---|---|---|---|---|
| | Before | After | Before | After | Before | After | Before | After | |
| __ / __ / __ | | | | | | | | | |

| Friday | Breakfast | | Lunch | | Dinner | | Bedtime | | Notes |
|---|---|---|---|---|---|---|---|---|---|
| | Before | After | Before | After | Before | After | Before | After | |
| __ / __ / __ | | | | | | | | | |

| Saturday | Breakfast | | Lunch | | Dinner | | Bedtime | | Notes |
|---|---|---|---|---|---|---|---|---|---|
| | Before | After | Before | After | Before | After | Before | After | |
| __ / __ / __ | | | | | | | | | |

| Sunday | Breakfast | | Lunch | | Dinner | | Bedtime | | Notes |
|---|---|---|---|---|---|---|---|---|---|
| | Before | After | Before | After | Before | After | Before | After | |
| __ / __ / __ | | | | | | | | | |

| Week: _____ | | | | | | | | | Weight: _____ |

| Monday | Breakfast | | Lunch | | Dinner | | Bedtime | | Notes |
|---|---|---|---|---|---|---|---|---|---|
| | Before | After | Before | After | Before | After | Before | After | |
| __/__/__ | | | | | | | | | |

| Tuesday | Breakfast | | Lunch | | Dinner | | Bedtime | | Notes |
|---|---|---|---|---|---|---|---|---|---|
| | Before | After | Before | After | Before | After | Before | After | |
| __/__/__ | | | | | | | | | |

| Wednesday | Breakfast | | Lunch | | Dinner | | Bedtime | | Notes |
|---|---|---|---|---|---|---|---|---|---|
| | Before | After | Before | After | Before | After | Before | After | |
| __/__/__ | | | | | | | | | |

| Thursday | Breakfast | | Lunch | | Dinner | | Bedtime | | Notes |
|---|---|---|---|---|---|---|---|---|---|
| | Before | After | Before | After | Before | After | Before | After | |
| __/__/__ | | | | | | | | | |

| Friday | Breakfast | | Lunch | | Dinner | | Bedtime | | Notes |
|---|---|---|---|---|---|---|---|---|---|
| | Before | After | Before | After | Before | After | Before | After | |
| __/__/__ | | | | | | | | | |

| Saturday | Breakfast | | Lunch | | Dinner | | Bedtime | | Notes |
|---|---|---|---|---|---|---|---|---|---|
| | Before | After | Before | After | Before | After | Before | After | |
| __/__/__ | | | | | | | | | |

| Sunday | Breakfast | | Lunch | | Dinner | | Bedtime | | Notes |
|---|---|---|---|---|---|---|---|---|---|
| | Before | After | Before | After | Before | After | Before | After | |
| __/__/__ | | | | | | | | | |

| Week: _____ | | | | | | | | | Weight: _____ |

| Monday | Breakfast | | Lunch | | Dinner | | Bedtime | | Notes |
|---|---|---|---|---|---|---|---|---|---|
| | Before | After | Before | After | Before | After | Before | After | |
| __ / __ / __ | | | | | | | | | |

| Tuesday | Breakfast | | Lunch | | Dinner | | Bedtime | | Notes |
|---|---|---|---|---|---|---|---|---|---|
| | Before | After | Before | After | Before | After | Before | After | |
| __ / __ / __ | | | | | | | | | |

| Wednesday | Breakfast | | Lunch | | Dinner | | Bedtime | | Notes |
|---|---|---|---|---|---|---|---|---|---|
| | Before | After | Before | After | Before | After | Before | After | |
| __ / __ / __ | | | | | | | | | |

| Thursday | Breakfast | | Lunch | | Dinner | | Bedtime | | Notes |
|---|---|---|---|---|---|---|---|---|---|
| | Before | After | Before | After | Before | After | Before | After | |
| __ / __ / __ | | | | | | | | | |

| Friday | Breakfast | | Lunch | | Dinner | | Bedtime | | Notes |
|---|---|---|---|---|---|---|---|---|---|
| | Before | After | Before | After | Before | After | Before | After | |
| __ / __ / __ | | | | | | | | | |

| Saturday | Breakfast | | Lunch | | Dinner | | Bedtime | | Notes |
|---|---|---|---|---|---|---|---|---|---|
| | Before | After | Before | After | Before | After | Before | After | |
| __ / __ / __ | | | | | | | | | |

| Sunday | Breakfast | | Lunch | | Dinner | | Bedtime | | Notes |
|---|---|---|---|---|---|---|---|---|---|
| | Before | After | Before | After | Before | After | Before | After | |
| __ / __ / __ | | | | | | | | | |

| Week: _____ | | | | | | | | | Weight: _____ |

| Monday | Breakfast | | Lunch | | Dinner | | Bedtime | | Notes |
|---|---|---|---|---|---|---|---|---|---|
| | Before | After | Before | After | Before | After | Before | After | |
| __ / __ / __ | | | | | | | | | |

| Tuesday | Breakfast | | Lunch | | Dinner | | Bedtime | | Notes |
|---|---|---|---|---|---|---|---|---|---|
| | Before | After | Before | After | Before | After | Before | After | |
| __ / __ / __ | | | | | | | | | |

| Wednesday | Breakfast | | Lunch | | Dinner | | Bedtime | | Notes |
|---|---|---|---|---|---|---|---|---|---|
| | Before | After | Before | After | Before | After | Before | After | |
| __ / __ / __ | | | | | | | | | |

| Thursday | Breakfast | | Lunch | | Dinner | | Bedtime | | Notes |
|---|---|---|---|---|---|---|---|---|---|
| | Before | After | Before | After | Before | After | Before | After | |
| __ / __ / __ | | | | | | | | | |

| Friday | Breakfast | | Lunch | | Dinner | | Bedtime | | Notes |
|---|---|---|---|---|---|---|---|---|---|
| | Before | After | Before | After | Before | After | Before | After | |
| __ / __ / __ | | | | | | | | | |

| Saturday | Breakfast | | Lunch | | Dinner | | Bedtime | | Notes |
|---|---|---|---|---|---|---|---|---|---|
| | Before | After | Before | After | Before | After | Before | After | |
| __ / __ / __ | | | | | | | | | |

| Sunday | Breakfast | | Lunch | | Dinner | | Bedtime | | Notes |
|---|---|---|---|---|---|---|---|---|---|
| | Before | After | Before | After | Before | After | Before | After | |
| __ / __ / __ | | | | | | | | | |

| Week: _____ | | | | | | | | | Weight: _____ |
|---|---|---|---|---|---|---|---|---|---|

| Monday | Breakfast | | Lunch | | Dinner | | Bedtime | | Notes |
|---|---|---|---|---|---|---|---|---|---|
| | Before | After | Before | After | Before | After | Before | After | |
| __ / __ / __ | | | | | | | | | |

| Tuesday | Breakfast | | Lunch | | Dinner | | Bedtime | | Notes |
|---|---|---|---|---|---|---|---|---|---|
| | Before | After | Before | After | Before | After | Before | After | |
| __ / __ / __ | | | | | | | | | |

| Wednesday | Breakfast | | Lunch | | Dinner | | Bedtime | | Notes |
|---|---|---|---|---|---|---|---|---|---|
| | Before | After | Before | After | Before | After | Before | After | |
| __ / __ / __ | | | | | | | | | |

| Thursday | Breakfast | | Lunch | | Dinner | | Bedtime | | Notes |
|---|---|---|---|---|---|---|---|---|---|
| | Before | After | Before | After | Before | After | Before | After | |
| __ / __ / __ | | | | | | | | | |

| Friday | Breakfast | | Lunch | | Dinner | | Bedtime | | Notes |
|---|---|---|---|---|---|---|---|---|---|
| | Before | After | Before | After | Before | After | Before | After | |
| __ / __ / __ | | | | | | | | | |

| Saturday | Breakfast | | Lunch | | Dinner | | Bedtime | | Notes |
|---|---|---|---|---|---|---|---|---|---|
| | Before | After | Before | After | Before | After | Before | After | |
| __ / __ / __ | | | | | | | | | |

| Sunday | Breakfast | | Lunch | | Dinner | | Bedtime | | Notes |
|---|---|---|---|---|---|---|---|---|---|
| | Before | After | Before | After | Before | After | Before | After | |
| __ / __ / __ | | | | | | | | | |

| Week: _____ | | | | | | | | | Weight: _____ |
|---|---|---|---|---|---|---|---|---|---|

| Monday | Breakfast | | Lunch | | Dinner | | Bedtime | | Notes |
|---|---|---|---|---|---|---|---|---|---|
| | Before | After | Before | After | Before | After | Before | After | |
| __/__/__ | | | | | | | | | |

| Tuesday | Breakfast | | Lunch | | Dinner | | Bedtime | | Notes |
|---|---|---|---|---|---|---|---|---|---|
| | Before | After | Before | After | Before | After | Before | After | |
| __/__/__ | | | | | | | | | |

| Wednesday | Breakfast | | Lunch | | Dinner | | Bedtime | | Notes |
|---|---|---|---|---|---|---|---|---|---|
| | Before | After | Before | After | Before | After | Before | After | |
| __/__/__ | | | | | | | | | |

| Thursday | Breakfast | | Lunch | | Dinner | | Bedtime | | Notes |
|---|---|---|---|---|---|---|---|---|---|
| | Before | After | Before | After | Before | After | Before | After | |
| __/__/__ | | | | | | | | | |

| Friday | Breakfast | | Lunch | | Dinner | | Bedtime | | Notes |
|---|---|---|---|---|---|---|---|---|---|
| | Before | After | Before | After | Before | After | Before | After | |
| __/__/__ | | | | | | | | | |

| Saturday | Breakfast | | Lunch | | Dinner | | Bedtime | | Notes |
|---|---|---|---|---|---|---|---|---|---|
| | Before | After | Before | After | Before | After | Before | After | |
| __/__/__ | | | | | | | | | |

| Sunday | Breakfast | | Lunch | | Dinner | | Bedtime | | Notes |
|---|---|---|---|---|---|---|---|---|---|
| | Before | After | Before | After | Before | After | Before | After | |
| __/__/__ | | | | | | | | | |

| Monday | Breakfast | | Lunch | | Dinner | | Bedtime | | Notes |
|---|---|---|---|---|---|---|---|---|---|
| | Before | After | Before | After | Before | After | Before | After | |
| __ / __ / __ | | | | | | | | | |

| Tuesday | Breakfast | | Lunch | | Dinner | | Bedtime | | Notes |
|---|---|---|---|---|---|---|---|---|---|
| | Before | After | Before | After | Before | After | Before | After | |
| __ / __ / __ | | | | | | | | | |

| Wednesday | Breakfast | | Lunch | | Dinner | | Bedtime | | Notes |
|---|---|---|---|---|---|---|---|---|---|
| | Before | After | Before | After | Before | After | Before | After | |
| __ / __ / __ | | | | | | | | | |

| Thursday | Breakfast | | Lunch | | Dinner | | Bedtime | | Notes |
|---|---|---|---|---|---|---|---|---|---|
| | Before | After | Before | After | Before | After | Before | After | |
| __ / __ / __ | | | | | | | | | |

| Friday | Breakfast | | Lunch | | Dinner | | Bedtime | | Notes |
|---|---|---|---|---|---|---|---|---|---|
| | Before | After | Before | After | Before | After | Before | After | |
| __ / __ / __ | | | | | | | | | |

| Saturday | Breakfast | | Lunch | | Dinner | | Bedtime | | Notes |
|---|---|---|---|---|---|---|---|---|---|
| | Before | After | Before | After | Before | After | Before | After | |
| __ / __ / __ | | | | | | | | | |

| Sunday | Breakfast | | Lunch | | Dinner | | Bedtime | | Notes |
|---|---|---|---|---|---|---|---|---|---|
| | Before | After | Before | After | Before | After | Before | After | |
| __ / __ / __ | | | | | | | | | |

| Week: _____ | | | | | | | | | Weight: _____ | |

| Monday | Breakfast | | Lunch | | Dinner | | Bedtime | | Notes |
|---|---|---|---|---|---|---|---|---|---|
| | Before | After | Before | After | Before | After | Before | After | |
| __/__/__ | | | | | | | | | |

| Tuesday | Breakfast | | Lunch | | Dinner | | Bedtime | | Notes |
|---|---|---|---|---|---|---|---|---|---|
| | Before | After | Before | After | Before | After | Before | After | |
| __/__/__ | | | | | | | | | |

| Wednesday | Breakfast | | Lunch | | Dinner | | Bedtime | | Notes |
|---|---|---|---|---|---|---|---|---|---|
| | Before | After | Before | After | Before | After | Before | After | |
| __/__/__ | | | | | | | | | |

| Thursday | Breakfast | | Lunch | | Dinner | | Bedtime | | Notes |
|---|---|---|---|---|---|---|---|---|---|
| | Before | After | Before | After | Before | After | Before | After | |
| __/__/__ | | | | | | | | | |

| Friday | Breakfast | | Lunch | | Dinner | | Bedtime | | Notes |
|---|---|---|---|---|---|---|---|---|---|
| | Before | After | Before | After | Before | After | Before | After | |
| __/__/__ | | | | | | | | | |

| Saturday | Breakfast | | Lunch | | Dinner | | Bedtime | | Notes |
|---|---|---|---|---|---|---|---|---|---|
| | Before | After | Before | After | Before | After | Before | After | |
| __/__/__ | | | | | | | | | |

| Sunday | Breakfast | | Lunch | | Dinner | | Bedtime | | Notes |
|---|---|---|---|---|---|---|---|---|---|
| | Before | After | Before | After | Before | After | Before | After | |
| __/__/__ | | | | | | | | | |

| Week: _____ | | | | | | | | | Weight: _____ |
|---|---|---|---|---|---|---|---|---|---|

| Monday | Breakfast | | Lunch | | Dinner | | Bedtime | | Notes |
|---|---|---|---|---|---|---|---|---|---|
| | Before | After | Before | After | Before | After | Before | After | |
| __ / __ / __ | | | | | | | | | |

| Tuesday | Breakfast | | Lunch | | Dinner | | Bedtime | | Notes |
|---|---|---|---|---|---|---|---|---|---|
| | Before | After | Before | After | Before | After | Before | After | |
| __ / __ / __ | | | | | | | | | |

| Wednesday | Breakfast | | Lunch | | Dinner | | Bedtime | | Notes |
|---|---|---|---|---|---|---|---|---|---|
| | Before | After | Before | After | Before | After | Before | After | |
| __ / __ / __ | | | | | | | | | |

| Thursday | Breakfast | | Lunch | | Dinner | | Bedtime | | Notes |
|---|---|---|---|---|---|---|---|---|---|
| | Before | After | Before | After | Before | After | Before | After | |
| __ / __ / __ | | | | | | | | | |

| Friday | Breakfast | | Lunch | | Dinner | | Bedtime | | Notes |
|---|---|---|---|---|---|---|---|---|---|
| | Before | After | Before | After | Before | After | Before | After | |
| __ / __ / __ | | | | | | | | | |

| Saturday | Breakfast | | Lunch | | Dinner | | Bedtime | | Notes |
|---|---|---|---|---|---|---|---|---|---|
| | Before | After | Before | After | Before | After | Before | After | |
| __ / __ / __ | | | | | | | | | |

| Sunday | Breakfast | | Lunch | | Dinner | | Bedtime | | Notes |
|---|---|---|---|---|---|---|---|---|---|
| | Before | After | Before | After | Before | After | Before | After | |
| __ / __ / __ | | | | | | | | | |

| Week: _____ | | | | | | | | | Weight: _____ |
|---|---|---|---|---|---|---|---|---|---|

| Monday | Breakfast | | Lunch | | Dinner | | Bedtime | | Notes |
|---|---|---|---|---|---|---|---|---|---|
| | Before | After | Before | After | Before | After | Before | After | |
| __/__/__ | | | | | | | | | |

| Tuesday | Breakfast | | Lunch | | Dinner | | Bedtime | | Notes |
|---|---|---|---|---|---|---|---|---|---|
| | Before | After | Before | After | Before | After | Before | After | |
| __/__/__ | | | | | | | | | |

| Wednesday | Breakfast | | Lunch | | Dinner | | Bedtime | | Notes |
|---|---|---|---|---|---|---|---|---|---|
| | Before | After | Before | After | Before | After | Before | After | |
| __/__/__ | | | | | | | | | |

| Thursday | Breakfast | | Lunch | | Dinner | | Bedtime | | Notes |
|---|---|---|---|---|---|---|---|---|---|
| | Before | After | Before | After | Before | After | Before | After | |
| __/__/__ | | | | | | | | | |

| Friday | Breakfast | | Lunch | | Dinner | | Bedtime | | Notes |
|---|---|---|---|---|---|---|---|---|---|
| | Before | After | Before | After | Before | After | Before | After | |
| __/__/__ | | | | | | | | | |

| Saturday | Breakfast | | Lunch | | Dinner | | Bedtime | | Notes |
|---|---|---|---|---|---|---|---|---|---|
| | Before | After | Before | After | Before | After | Before | After | |
| __/__/__ | | | | | | | | | |

| Sunday | Breakfast | | Lunch | | Dinner | | Bedtime | | Notes |
|---|---|---|---|---|---|---|---|---|---|
| | Before | After | Before | After | Before | After | Before | After | |
| __/__/__ | | | | | | | | | |

<table>
<tr><td rowspan="2">Week: _____</td><td colspan="8"></td><td rowspan="2">Weight: _____</td></tr>
</table>

| Monday __/__/__ | Breakfast | | Lunch | | Dinner | | Bedtime | | Notes |
|---|---|---|---|---|---|---|---|---|---|
| | Before | After | Before | After | Before | After | Before | After | |
| | | | | | | | | | |

| Tuesday __/__/__ | Breakfast | | Lunch | | Dinner | | Bedtime | | Notes |
|---|---|---|---|---|---|---|---|---|---|
| | Before | After | Before | After | Before | After | Before | After | |
| | | | | | | | | | |

| Wednesday __/__/__ | Breakfast | | Lunch | | Dinner | | Bedtime | | Notes |
|---|---|---|---|---|---|---|---|---|---|
| | Before | After | Before | After | Before | After | Before | After | |
| | | | | | | | | | |

| Thursday __/__/__ | Breakfast | | Lunch | | Dinner | | Bedtime | | Notes |
|---|---|---|---|---|---|---|---|---|---|
| | Before | After | Before | After | Before | After | Before | After | |
| | | | | | | | | | |

| Friday __/__/__ | Breakfast | | Lunch | | Dinner | | Bedtime | | Notes |
|---|---|---|---|---|---|---|---|---|---|
| | Before | After | Before | After | Before | After | Before | After | |
| | | | | | | | | | |

| Saturday __/__/__ | Breakfast | | Lunch | | Dinner | | Bedtime | | Notes |
|---|---|---|---|---|---|---|---|---|---|
| | Before | After | Before | After | Before | After | Before | After | |
| | | | | | | | | | |

| Sunday __/__/__ | Breakfast | | Lunch | | Dinner | | Bedtime | | Notes |
|---|---|---|---|---|---|---|---|---|---|
| | Before | After | Before | After | Before | After | Before | After | |
| | | | | | | | | | |

| Week: _____ | | | | | | | | | Weight: _____ |

| Monday | Breakfast | | Lunch | | Dinner | | Bedtime | | Notes |
|---|---|---|---|---|---|---|---|---|---|
| | Before | After | Before | After | Before | After | Before | After | |
| __/__/__ | | | | | | | | | |

| Tuesday | Breakfast | | Lunch | | Dinner | | Bedtime | | Notes |
|---|---|---|---|---|---|---|---|---|---|
| | Before | After | Before | After | Before | After | Before | After | |
| __/__/__ | | | | | | | | | |

| Wednesday | Breakfast | | Lunch | | Dinner | | Bedtime | | Notes |
|---|---|---|---|---|---|---|---|---|---|
| | Before | After | Before | After | Before | After | Before | After | |
| __/__/__ | | | | | | | | | |

| Thursday | Breakfast | | Lunch | | Dinner | | Bedtime | | Notes |
|---|---|---|---|---|---|---|---|---|---|
| | Before | After | Before | After | Before | After | Before | After | |
| __/__/__ | | | | | | | | | |

| Friday | Breakfast | | Lunch | | Dinner | | Bedtime | | Notes |
|---|---|---|---|---|---|---|---|---|---|
| | Before | After | Before | After | Before | After | Before | After | |
| __/__/__ | | | | | | | | | |

| Saturday | Breakfast | | Lunch | | Dinner | | Bedtime | | Notes |
|---|---|---|---|---|---|---|---|---|---|
| | Before | After | Before | After | Before | After | Before | After | |
| __/__/__ | | | | | | | | | |

| Sunday | Breakfast | | Lunch | | Dinner | | Bedtime | | Notes |
|---|---|---|---|---|---|---|---|---|---|
| | Before | After | Before | After | Before | After | Before | After | |
| __/__/__ | | | | | | | | | |

| Week: _____ | | | | | | | | | Weight: _____ |

| Monday __/__/__ | Breakfast | | Lunch | | Dinner | | Bedtime | | Notes |
|---|---|---|---|---|---|---|---|---|---|
| | Before | After | Before | After | Before | After | Before | After | |
| | | | | | | | | | |

| Tuesday __/__/__ | Breakfast | | Lunch | | Dinner | | Bedtime | | Notes |
|---|---|---|---|---|---|---|---|---|---|
| | Before | After | Before | After | Before | After | Before | After | |
| | | | | | | | | | |

| Wednesday __/__/__ | Breakfast | | Lunch | | Dinner | | Bedtime | | Notes |
|---|---|---|---|---|---|---|---|---|---|
| | Before | After | Before | After | Before | After | Before | After | |
| | | | | | | | | | |

| Thursday __/__/__ | Breakfast | | Lunch | | Dinner | | Bedtime | | Notes |
|---|---|---|---|---|---|---|---|---|---|
| | Before | After | Before | After | Before | After | Before | After | |
| | | | | | | | | | |

| Friday __/__/__ | Breakfast | | Lunch | | Dinner | | Bedtime | | Notes |
|---|---|---|---|---|---|---|---|---|---|
| | Before | After | Before | After | Before | After | Before | After | |
| | | | | | | | | | |

| Saturday __/__/__ | Breakfast | | Lunch | | Dinner | | Bedtime | | Notes |
|---|---|---|---|---|---|---|---|---|---|
| | Before | After | Before | After | Before | After | Before | After | |
| | | | | | | | | | |

| Sunday __/__/__ | Breakfast | | Lunch | | Dinner | | Bedtime | | Notes |
|---|---|---|---|---|---|---|---|---|---|
| | Before | After | Before | After | Before | After | Before | After | |
| | | | | | | | | | |

| Week: _____ | | | | | | | | | Weight: _____ |

| Monday | Breakfast | | Lunch | | Dinner | | Bedtime | | Notes |
|---|---|---|---|---|---|---|---|---|---|
| | Before | After | Before | After | Before | After | Before | After | |
| __/__/__ | | | | | | | | | |

| Tuesday | Breakfast | | Lunch | | Dinner | | Bedtime | | Notes |
|---|---|---|---|---|---|---|---|---|---|
| | Before | After | Before | After | Before | After | Before | After | |
| __/__/__ | | | | | | | | | |

| Wednesday | Breakfast | | Lunch | | Dinner | | Bedtime | | Notes |
|---|---|---|---|---|---|---|---|---|---|
| | Before | After | Before | After | Before | After | Before | After | |
| __/__/__ | | | | | | | | | |

| Thursday | Breakfast | | Lunch | | Dinner | | Bedtime | | Notes |
|---|---|---|---|---|---|---|---|---|---|
| | Before | After | Before | After | Before | After | Before | After | |
| __/__/__ | | | | | | | | | |

| Friday | Breakfast | | Lunch | | Dinner | | Bedtime | | Notes |
|---|---|---|---|---|---|---|---|---|---|
| | Before | After | Before | After | Before | After | Before | After | |
| __/__/__ | | | | | | | | | |

| Saturday | Breakfast | | Lunch | | Dinner | | Bedtime | | Notes |
|---|---|---|---|---|---|---|---|---|---|
| | Before | After | Before | After | Before | After | Before | After | |
| __/__/__ | | | | | | | | | |

| Sunday | Breakfast | | Lunch | | Dinner | | Bedtime | | Notes |
|---|---|---|---|---|---|---|---|---|---|
| | Before | After | Before | After | Before | After | Before | After | |
| __/__/__ | | | | | | | | | |

| Week: _____ | | | | | | | | | Weight: _____ |

| Monday | Breakfast | | Lunch | | Dinner | | Bedtime | | Notes |
|---|---|---|---|---|---|---|---|---|---|
| | Before | After | Before | After | Before | After | Before | After | |
| __ / __ / __ | | | | | | | | | |

| Tuesday | Breakfast | | Lunch | | Dinner | | Bedtime | | Notes |
|---|---|---|---|---|---|---|---|---|---|
| | Before | After | Before | After | Before | After | Before | After | |
| __ / __ / __ | | | | | | | | | |

| Wednesday | Breakfast | | Lunch | | Dinner | | Bedtime | | Notes |
|---|---|---|---|---|---|---|---|---|---|
| | Before | After | Before | After | Before | After | Before | After | |
| __ / __ / __ | | | | | | | | | |

| Thursday | Breakfast | | Lunch | | Dinner | | Bedtime | | Notes |
|---|---|---|---|---|---|---|---|---|---|
| | Before | After | Before | After | Before | After | Before | After | |
| __ / __ / __ | | | | | | | | | |

| Friday | Breakfast | | Lunch | | Dinner | | Bedtime | | Notes |
|---|---|---|---|---|---|---|---|---|---|
| | Before | After | Before | After | Before | After | Before | After | |
| __ / __ / __ | | | | | | | | | |

| Saturday | Breakfast | | Lunch | | Dinner | | Bedtime | | Notes |
|---|---|---|---|---|---|---|---|---|---|
| | Before | After | Before | After | Before | After | Before | After | |
| __ / __ / __ | | | | | | | | | |

| Sunday | Breakfast | | Lunch | | Dinner | | Bedtime | | Notes |
|---|---|---|---|---|---|---|---|---|---|
| | Before | After | Before | After | Before | After | Before | After | |
| __ / __ / __ | | | | | | | | | |

| Monday __/__/__ | Breakfast | | Lunch | | Dinner | | Bedtime | | Notes |
|---|---|---|---|---|---|---|---|---|---|
| | Before | After | Before | After | Before | After | Before | After | |
| | | | | | | | | | |

| Tuesday __/__/__ | Breakfast | | Lunch | | Dinner | | Bedtime | | Notes |
|---|---|---|---|---|---|---|---|---|---|
| | Before | After | Before | After | Before | After | Before | After | |
| | | | | | | | | | |

| Wednesday __/__/__ | Breakfast | | Lunch | | Dinner | | Bedtime | | Notes |
|---|---|---|---|---|---|---|---|---|---|
| | Before | After | Before | After | Before | After | Before | After | |
| | | | | | | | | | |

| Thursday __/__/__ | Breakfast | | Lunch | | Dinner | | Bedtime | | Notes |
|---|---|---|---|---|---|---|---|---|---|
| | Before | After | Before | After | Before | After | Before | After | |
| | | | | | | | | | |

| Friday __/__/__ | Breakfast | | Lunch | | Dinner | | Bedtime | | Notes |
|---|---|---|---|---|---|---|---|---|---|
| | Before | After | Before | After | Before | After | Before | After | |
| | | | | | | | | | |

| Saturday __/__/__ | Breakfast | | Lunch | | Dinner | | Bedtime | | Notes |
|---|---|---|---|---|---|---|---|---|---|
| | Before | After | Before | After | Before | After | Before | After | |
| | | | | | | | | | |

| Sunday __/__/__ | Breakfast | | Lunch | | Dinner | | Bedtime | | Notes |
|---|---|---|---|---|---|---|---|---|---|
| | Before | After | Before | After | Before | After | Before | After | |
| | | | | | | | | | |

| Week: _____ | | | | | | | | | Weight: _____ |
|---|---|---|---|---|---|---|---|---|---|

| Monday | Breakfast | | Lunch | | Dinner | | Bedtime | | Notes |
|---|---|---|---|---|---|---|---|---|---|
| | Before | After | Before | After | Before | After | Before | After | |
| __ / __ / __ | | | | | | | | | |

| Tuesday | Breakfast | | Lunch | | Dinner | | Bedtime | | Notes |
|---|---|---|---|---|---|---|---|---|---|
| | Before | After | Before | After | Before | After | Before | After | |
| __ / __ / __ | | | | | | | | | |

| Wednesday | Breakfast | | Lunch | | Dinner | | Bedtime | | Notes |
|---|---|---|---|---|---|---|---|---|---|
| | Before | After | Before | After | Before | After | Before | After | |
| __ / __ / __ | | | | | | | | | |

| Thursday | Breakfast | | Lunch | | Dinner | | Bedtime | | Notes |
|---|---|---|---|---|---|---|---|---|---|
| | Before | After | Before | After | Before | After | Before | After | |
| __ / __ / __ | | | | | | | | | |

| Friday | Breakfast | | Lunch | | Dinner | | Bedtime | | Notes |
|---|---|---|---|---|---|---|---|---|---|
| | Before | After | Before | After | Before | After | Before | After | |
| __ / __ / __ | | | | | | | | | |

| Saturday | Breakfast | | Lunch | | Dinner | | Bedtime | | Notes |
|---|---|---|---|---|---|---|---|---|---|
| | Before | After | Before | After | Before | After | Before | After | |
| __ / __ / __ | | | | | | | | | |

| Sunday | Breakfast | | Lunch | | Dinner | | Bedtime | | Notes |
|---|---|---|---|---|---|---|---|---|---|
| | Before | After | Before | After | Before | After | Before | After | |
| __ / __ / __ | | | | | | | | | |

<table>
<tr><td>Week: _____</td><td colspan="8"></td><td>Weight: _____</td></tr>
</table>

| Monday __/__/__ | Breakfast | | Lunch | | Dinner | | Bedtime | | Notes |
|---|---|---|---|---|---|---|---|---|---|
| | Before | After | Before | After | Before | After | Before | After | |
| | | | | | | | | | |

| Tuesday __/__/__ | Breakfast | | Lunch | | Dinner | | Bedtime | | Notes |
|---|---|---|---|---|---|---|---|---|---|
| | Before | After | Before | After | Before | After | Before | After | |
| | | | | | | | | | |

| Wednesday __/__/__ | Breakfast | | Lunch | | Dinner | | Bedtime | | Notes |
|---|---|---|---|---|---|---|---|---|---|
| | Before | After | Before | After | Before | After | Before | After | |
| | | | | | | | | | |

| Thursday __/__/__ | Breakfast | | Lunch | | Dinner | | Bedtime | | Notes |
|---|---|---|---|---|---|---|---|---|---|
| | Before | After | Before | After | Before | After | Before | After | |
| | | | | | | | | | |

| Friday __/__/__ | Breakfast | | Lunch | | Dinner | | Bedtime | | Notes |
|---|---|---|---|---|---|---|---|---|---|
| | Before | After | Before | After | Before | After | Before | After | |
| | | | | | | | | | |

| Saturday __/__/__ | Breakfast | | Lunch | | Dinner | | Bedtime | | Notes |
|---|---|---|---|---|---|---|---|---|---|
| | Before | After | Before | After | Before | After | Before | After | |
| | | | | | | | | | |

| Sunday __/__/__ | Breakfast | | Lunch | | Dinner | | Bedtime | | Notes |
|---|---|---|---|---|---|---|---|---|---|
| | Before | After | Before | After | Before | After | Before | After | |
| | | | | | | | | | |

| Week: _____ | | | | | | | | | Weight: _____ |

| Monday | Breakfast | | Lunch | | Dinner | | Bedtime | | Notes |
|---|---|---|---|---|---|---|---|---|---|
| | Before | After | Before | After | Before | After | Before | After | |
| __ / __ / __ | | | | | | | | | |

| Tuesday | Breakfast | | Lunch | | Dinner | | Bedtime | | Notes |
|---|---|---|---|---|---|---|---|---|---|
| | Before | After | Before | After | Before | After | Before | After | |
| __ / __ / __ | | | | | | | | | |

| Wednesday | Breakfast | | Lunch | | Dinner | | Bedtime | | Notes |
|---|---|---|---|---|---|---|---|---|---|
| | Before | After | Before | After | Before | After | Before | After | |
| __ / __ / __ | | | | | | | | | |

| Thursday | Breakfast | | Lunch | | Dinner | | Bedtime | | Notes |
|---|---|---|---|---|---|---|---|---|---|
| | Before | After | Before | After | Before | After | Before | After | |
| __ / __ / __ | | | | | | | | | |

| Friday | Breakfast | | Lunch | | Dinner | | Bedtime | | Notes |
|---|---|---|---|---|---|---|---|---|---|
| | Before | After | Before | After | Before | After | Before | After | |
| __ / __ / __ | | | | | | | | | |

| Saturday | Breakfast | | Lunch | | Dinner | | Bedtime | | Notes |
|---|---|---|---|---|---|---|---|---|---|
| | Before | After | Before | After | Before | After | Before | After | |
| __ / __ / __ | | | | | | | | | |

| Sunday | Breakfast | | Lunch | | Dinner | | Bedtime | | Notes |
|---|---|---|---|---|---|---|---|---|---|
| | Before | After | Before | After | Before | After | Before | After | |
| __ / __ / __ | | | | | | | | | |

| Week: _____ | | | | | | | | | Weight: _____ |
|---|---|---|---|---|---|---|---|---|---|

| Monday | Breakfast | | Lunch | | Dinner | | Bedtime | | Notes |
|---|---|---|---|---|---|---|---|---|---|
| | Before | After | Before | After | Before | After | Before | After | |
| __ / __ / __ | | | | | | | | | |

| Tuesday | Breakfast | | Lunch | | Dinner | | Bedtime | | Notes |
|---|---|---|---|---|---|---|---|---|---|
| | Before | After | Before | After | Before | After | Before | After | |
| __ / __ / __ | | | | | | | | | |

| Wednesday | Breakfast | | Lunch | | Dinner | | Bedtime | | Notes |
|---|---|---|---|---|---|---|---|---|---|
| | Before | After | Before | After | Before | After | Before | After | |
| __ / __ / __ | | | | | | | | | |

| Thursday | Breakfast | | Lunch | | Dinner | | Bedtime | | Notes |
|---|---|---|---|---|---|---|---|---|---|
| | Before | After | Before | After | Before | After | Before | After | |
| __ / __ / __ | | | | | | | | | |

| Friday | Breakfast | | Lunch | | Dinner | | Bedtime | | Notes |
|---|---|---|---|---|---|---|---|---|---|
| | Before | After | Before | After | Before | After | Before | After | |
| __ / __ / __ | | | | | | | | | |

| Saturday | Breakfast | | Lunch | | Dinner | | Bedtime | | Notes |
|---|---|---|---|---|---|---|---|---|---|
| | Before | After | Before | After | Before | After | Before | After | |
| __ / __ / __ | | | | | | | | | |

| Sunday | Breakfast | | Lunch | | Dinner | | Bedtime | | Notes |
|---|---|---|---|---|---|---|---|---|---|
| | Before | After | Before | After | Before | After | Before | After | |
| __ / __ / __ | | | | | | | | | |

| Monday | Breakfast | | Lunch | | Dinner | | Bedtime | | Notes |
|---|---|---|---|---|---|---|---|---|---|
| | Before | After | Before | After | Before | After | Before | After | |
| __ / __ / __ | | | | | | | | | |

| Tuesday | Breakfast | | Lunch | | Dinner | | Bedtime | | Notes |
|---|---|---|---|---|---|---|---|---|---|
| | Before | After | Before | After | Before | After | Before | After | |
| __ / __ / __ | | | | | | | | | |

| Wednesday | Breakfast | | Lunch | | Dinner | | Bedtime | | Notes |
|---|---|---|---|---|---|---|---|---|---|
| | Before | After | Before | After | Before | After | Before | After | |
| __ / __ / __ | | | | | | | | | |

| Thursday | Breakfast | | Lunch | | Dinner | | Bedtime | | Notes |
|---|---|---|---|---|---|---|---|---|---|
| | Before | After | Before | After | Before | After | Before | After | |
| __ / __ / __ | | | | | | | | | |

| Friday | Breakfast | | Lunch | | Dinner | | Bedtime | | Notes |
|---|---|---|---|---|---|---|---|---|---|
| | Before | After | Before | After | Before | After | Before | After | |
| __ / __ / __ | | | | | | | | | |

| Saturday | Breakfast | | Lunch | | Dinner | | Bedtime | | Notes |
|---|---|---|---|---|---|---|---|---|---|
| | Before | After | Before | After | Before | After | Before | After | |
| __ / __ / __ | | | | | | | | | |

| Sunday | Breakfast | | Lunch | | Dinner | | Bedtime | | Notes |
|---|---|---|---|---|---|---|---|---|---|
| | Before | After | Before | After | Before | After | Before | After | |
| __ / __ / __ | | | | | | | | | |

| Week: _____ | | | | | Weight: _____ |

| Monday | Breakfast | | Lunch | | Dinner | | Bedtime | | Notes |
|---|---|---|---|---|---|---|---|---|---|
| | Before | After | Before | After | Before | After | Before | After | |
| __ / __ / __ | | | | | | | | | |

| Tuesday | Breakfast | | Lunch | | Dinner | | Bedtime | | Notes |
|---|---|---|---|---|---|---|---|---|---|
| | Before | After | Before | After | Before | After | Before | After | |
| __ / __ / __ | | | | | | | | | |

| Wednesday | Breakfast | | Lunch | | Dinner | | Bedtime | | Notes |
|---|---|---|---|---|---|---|---|---|---|
| | Before | After | Before | After | Before | After | Before | After | |
| __ / __ / __ | | | | | | | | | |

| Thursday | Breakfast | | Lunch | | Dinner | | Bedtime | | Notes |
|---|---|---|---|---|---|---|---|---|---|
| | Before | After | Before | After | Before | After | Before | After | |
| __ / __ / __ | | | | | | | | | |

| Friday | Breakfast | | Lunch | | Dinner | | Bedtime | | Notes |
|---|---|---|---|---|---|---|---|---|---|
| | Before | After | Before | After | Before | After | Before | After | |
| __ / __ / __ | | | | | | | | | |

| Saturday | Breakfast | | Lunch | | Dinner | | Bedtime | | Notes |
|---|---|---|---|---|---|---|---|---|---|
| | Before | After | Before | After | Before | After | Before | After | |
| __ / __ / __ | | | | | | | | | |

| Sunday | Breakfast | | Lunch | | Dinner | | Bedtime | | Notes |
|---|---|---|---|---|---|---|---|---|---|
| | Before | After | Before | After | Before | After | Before | After | |
| __ / __ / __ | | | | | | | | | |

| Week: _____ | | | | | | | | | Weight: _____ |
|---|---|---|---|---|---|---|---|---|---|

| Monday | Breakfast | | Lunch | | Dinner | | Bedtime | | Notes |
|---|---|---|---|---|---|---|---|---|---|
| | Before | After | Before | After | Before | After | Before | After | |
| __/__/__ | | | | | | | | | |

| Tuesday | Breakfast | | Lunch | | Dinner | | Bedtime | | Notes |
|---|---|---|---|---|---|---|---|---|---|
| | Before | After | Before | After | Before | After | Before | After | |
| __/__/__ | | | | | | | | | |

| Wednesday | Breakfast | | Lunch | | Dinner | | Bedtime | | Notes |
|---|---|---|---|---|---|---|---|---|---|
| | Before | After | Before | After | Before | After | Before | After | |
| __/__/__ | | | | | | | | | |

| Thursday | Breakfast | | Lunch | | Dinner | | Bedtime | | Notes |
|---|---|---|---|---|---|---|---|---|---|
| | Before | After | Before | After | Before | After | Before | After | |
| __/__/__ | | | | | | | | | |

| Friday | Breakfast | | Lunch | | Dinner | | Bedtime | | Notes |
|---|---|---|---|---|---|---|---|---|---|
| | Before | After | Before | After | Before | After | Before | After | |
| __/__/__ | | | | | | | | | |

| Saturday | Breakfast | | Lunch | | Dinner | | Bedtime | | Notes |
|---|---|---|---|---|---|---|---|---|---|
| | Before | After | Before | After | Before | After | Before | After | |
| __/__/__ | | | | | | | | | |

| Sunday | Breakfast | | Lunch | | Dinner | | Bedtime | | Notes |
|---|---|---|---|---|---|---|---|---|---|
| | Before | After | Before | After | Before | After | Before | After | |
| __/__/__ | | | | | | | | | |

**Week:** _____      **Weight:** _____

| Monday | Breakfast | | Lunch | | Dinner | | Bedtime | | Notes |
|---|---|---|---|---|---|---|---|---|---|
| | Before | After | Before | After | Before | After | Before | After | |
| __ / __ / __ | | | | | | | | | |

| Tuesday | Breakfast | | Lunch | | Dinner | | Bedtime | | Notes |
|---|---|---|---|---|---|---|---|---|---|
| | Before | After | Before | After | Before | After | Before | After | |
| __ / __ / __ | | | | | | | | | |

| Wednesday | Breakfast | | Lunch | | Dinner | | Bedtime | | Notes |
|---|---|---|---|---|---|---|---|---|---|
| | Before | After | Before | After | Before | After | Before | After | |
| __ / __ / __ | | | | | | | | | |

| Thursday | Breakfast | | Lunch | | Dinner | | Bedtime | | Notes |
|---|---|---|---|---|---|---|---|---|---|
| | Before | After | Before | After | Before | After | Before | After | |
| __ / __ / __ | | | | | | | | | |

| Friday | Breakfast | | Lunch | | Dinner | | Bedtime | | Notes |
|---|---|---|---|---|---|---|---|---|---|
| | Before | After | Before | After | Before | After | Before | After | |
| __ / __ / __ | | | | | | | | | |

| Saturday | Breakfast | | Lunch | | Dinner | | Bedtime | | Notes |
|---|---|---|---|---|---|---|---|---|---|
| | Before | After | Before | After | Before | After | Before | After | |
| __ / __ / __ | | | | | | | | | |

| Sunday | Breakfast | | Lunch | | Dinner | | Bedtime | | Notes |
|---|---|---|---|---|---|---|---|---|---|
| | Before | After | Before | After | Before | After | Before | After | |
| __ / __ / __ | | | | | | | | | |

| Week: _____ | | | | | | | | | Weight: _____ |
|---|---|---|---|---|---|---|---|---|---|

| Monday | Breakfast | | Lunch | | Dinner | | Bedtime | | Notes |
|---|---|---|---|---|---|---|---|---|---|
| | Before | After | Before | After | Before | After | Before | After | |
| __ / __ / __ | | | | | | | | | |

| Tuesday | Breakfast | | Lunch | | Dinner | | Bedtime | | Notes |
|---|---|---|---|---|---|---|---|---|---|
| | Before | After | Before | After | Before | After | Before | After | |
| __ / __ / __ | | | | | | | | | |

| Wednesday | Breakfast | | Lunch | | Dinner | | Bedtime | | Notes |
|---|---|---|---|---|---|---|---|---|---|
| | Before | After | Before | After | Before | After | Before | After | |
| __ / __ / __ | | | | | | | | | |

| Thursday | Breakfast | | Lunch | | Dinner | | Bedtime | | Notes |
|---|---|---|---|---|---|---|---|---|---|
| | Before | After | Before | After | Before | After | Before | After | |
| __ / __ / __ | | | | | | | | | |

| Friday | Breakfast | | Lunch | | Dinner | | Bedtime | | Notes |
|---|---|---|---|---|---|---|---|---|---|
| | Before | After | Before | After | Before | After | Before | After | |
| __ / __ / __ | | | | | | | | | |

| Saturday | Breakfast | | Lunch | | Dinner | | Bedtime | | Notes |
|---|---|---|---|---|---|---|---|---|---|
| | Before | After | Before | After | Before | After | Before | After | |
| __ / __ / __ | | | | | | | | | |

| Sunday | Breakfast | | Lunch | | Dinner | | Bedtime | | Notes |
|---|---|---|---|---|---|---|---|---|---|
| | Before | After | Before | After | Before | After | Before | After | |
| __ / __ / __ | | | | | | | | | |

| Week: _____ | | | | | | | | | Weight: _____ |
|---|---|---|---|---|---|---|---|---|---|

| Monday | Breakfast | | Lunch | | Dinner | | Bedtime | | Notes |
|---|---|---|---|---|---|---|---|---|---|
| | Before | After | Before | After | Before | After | Before | After | |
| __/__/__ | | | | | | | | | |

| Tuesday | Breakfast | | Lunch | | Dinner | | Bedtime | | Notes |
|---|---|---|---|---|---|---|---|---|---|
| | Before | After | Before | After | Before | After | Before | After | |
| __/__/__ | | | | | | | | | |

| Wednesday | Breakfast | | Lunch | | Dinner | | Bedtime | | Notes |
|---|---|---|---|---|---|---|---|---|---|
| | Before | After | Before | After | Before | After | Before | After | |
| __/__/__ | | | | | | | | | |

| Thursday | Breakfast | | Lunch | | Dinner | | Bedtime | | Notes |
|---|---|---|---|---|---|---|---|---|---|
| | Before | After | Before | After | Before | After | Before | After | |
| __/__/__ | | | | | | | | | |

| Friday | Breakfast | | Lunch | | Dinner | | Bedtime | | Notes |
|---|---|---|---|---|---|---|---|---|---|
| | Before | After | Before | After | Before | After | Before | After | |
| __/__/__ | | | | | | | | | |

| Saturday | Breakfast | | Lunch | | Dinner | | Bedtime | | Notes |
|---|---|---|---|---|---|---|---|---|---|
| | Before | After | Before | After | Before | After | Before | After | |
| __/__/__ | | | | | | | | | |

| Sunday | Breakfast | | Lunch | | Dinner | | Bedtime | | Notes |
|---|---|---|---|---|---|---|---|---|---|
| | Before | After | Before | After | Before | After | Before | After | |
| __/__/__ | | | | | | | | | |

| Week: _____ | | | | | | | | Weight: _____ | |
|---|---|---|---|---|---|---|---|---|---|

| Monday | Breakfast | | Lunch | | Dinner | | Bedtime | | Notes |
|---|---|---|---|---|---|---|---|---|---|
| | Before | After | Before | After | Before | After | Before | After | |
| __/__/__ | | | | | | | | | |

| Tuesday | Breakfast | | Lunch | | Dinner | | Bedtime | | Notes |
|---|---|---|---|---|---|---|---|---|---|
| | Before | After | Before | After | Before | After | Before | After | |
| __/__/__ | | | | | | | | | |

| Wednesday | Breakfast | | Lunch | | Dinner | | Bedtime | | Notes |
|---|---|---|---|---|---|---|---|---|---|
| | Before | After | Before | After | Before | After | Before | After | |
| __/__/__ | | | | | | | | | |

| Thursday | Breakfast | | Lunch | | Dinner | | Bedtime | | Notes |
|---|---|---|---|---|---|---|---|---|---|
| | Before | After | Before | After | Before | After | Before | After | |
| __/__/__ | | | | | | | | | |

| Friday | Breakfast | | Lunch | | Dinner | | Bedtime | | Notes |
|---|---|---|---|---|---|---|---|---|---|
| | Before | After | Before | After | Before | After | Before | After | |
| __/__/__ | | | | | | | | | |

| Saturday | Breakfast | | Lunch | | Dinner | | Bedtime | | Notes |
|---|---|---|---|---|---|---|---|---|---|
| | Before | After | Before | After | Before | After | Before | After | |
| __/__/__ | | | | | | | | | |

| Sunday | Breakfast | | Lunch | | Dinner | | Bedtime | | Notes |
|---|---|---|---|---|---|---|---|---|---|
| | Before | After | Before | After | Before | After | Before | After | |
| __/__/__ | | | | | | | | | |

| Week: _____ | | | | | | | | | Weight: _____ |

| Monday | Breakfast | | Lunch | | Dinner | | Bedtime | | Notes |
|---|---|---|---|---|---|---|---|---|---|
| | Before | After | Before | After | Before | After | Before | After | |
| __/__/__ | | | | | | | | | |

| Tuesday | Breakfast | | Lunch | | Dinner | | Bedtime | | Notes |
|---|---|---|---|---|---|---|---|---|---|
| | Before | After | Before | After | Before | After | Before | After | |
| __/__/__ | | | | | | | | | |

| Wednesday | Breakfast | | Lunch | | Dinner | | Bedtime | | Notes |
|---|---|---|---|---|---|---|---|---|---|
| | Before | After | Before | After | Before | After | Before | After | |
| __/__/__ | | | | | | | | | |

| Thursday | Breakfast | | Lunch | | Dinner | | Bedtime | | Notes |
|---|---|---|---|---|---|---|---|---|---|
| | Before | After | Before | After | Before | After | Before | After | |
| __/__/__ | | | | | | | | | |

| Friday | Breakfast | | Lunch | | Dinner | | Bedtime | | Notes |
|---|---|---|---|---|---|---|---|---|---|
| | Before | After | Before | After | Before | After | Before | After | |
| __/__/__ | | | | | | | | | |

| Saturday | Breakfast | | Lunch | | Dinner | | Bedtime | | Notes |
|---|---|---|---|---|---|---|---|---|---|
| | Before | After | Before | After | Before | After | Before | After | |
| __/__/__ | | | | | | | | | |

| Sunday | Breakfast | | Lunch | | Dinner | | Bedtime | | Notes |
|---|---|---|---|---|---|---|---|---|---|
| | Before | After | Before | After | Before | After | Before | After | |
| __/__/__ | | | | | | | | | |

| Week: _____ | | | | | | | | | Weight: _____ |

| Monday | Breakfast | | Lunch | | Dinner | | Bedtime | | Notes |
|---|---|---|---|---|---|---|---|---|---|
| | Before | After | Before | After | Before | After | Before | After | |
| __ / __ / __ | | | | | | | | | |

| Tuesday | Breakfast | | Lunch | | Dinner | | Bedtime | | Notes |
|---|---|---|---|---|---|---|---|---|---|
| | Before | After | Before | After | Before | After | Before | After | |
| __ / __ / __ | | | | | | | | | |

| Wednesday | Breakfast | | Lunch | | Dinner | | Bedtime | | Notes |
|---|---|---|---|---|---|---|---|---|---|
| | Before | After | Before | After | Before | After | Before | After | |
| __ / __ / __ | | | | | | | | | |

| Thursday | Breakfast | | Lunch | | Dinner | | Bedtime | | Notes |
|---|---|---|---|---|---|---|---|---|---|
| | Before | After | Before | After | Before | After | Before | After | |
| __ / __ / __ | | | | | | | | | |

| Friday | Breakfast | | Lunch | | Dinner | | Bedtime | | Notes |
|---|---|---|---|---|---|---|---|---|---|
| | Before | After | Before | After | Before | After | Before | After | |
| __ / __ / __ | | | | | | | | | |

| Saturday | Breakfast | | Lunch | | Dinner | | Bedtime | | Notes |
|---|---|---|---|---|---|---|---|---|---|
| | Before | After | Before | After | Before | After | Before | After | |
| __ / __ / __ | | | | | | | | | |

| Sunday | Breakfast | | Lunch | | Dinner | | Bedtime | | Notes |
|---|---|---|---|---|---|---|---|---|---|
| | Before | After | Before | After | Before | After | Before | After | |
| __ / __ / __ | | | | | | | | | |

| Monday | Breakfast | | Lunch | | Dinner | | Bedtime | | Notes |
|---|---|---|---|---|---|---|---|---|---|
| | Before | After | Before | After | Before | After | Before | After | |
| __ / __ / __ | | | | | | | | | |

| Tuesday | Breakfast | | Lunch | | Dinner | | Bedtime | | Notes |
|---|---|---|---|---|---|---|---|---|---|
| | Before | After | Before | After | Before | After | Before | After | |
| __ / __ / __ | | | | | | | | | |

| Wednesday | Breakfast | | Lunch | | Dinner | | Bedtime | | Notes |
|---|---|---|---|---|---|---|---|---|---|
| | Before | After | Before | After | Before | After | Before | After | |
| __ / __ / __ | | | | | | | | | |

| Thursday | Breakfast | | Lunch | | Dinner | | Bedtime | | Notes |
|---|---|---|---|---|---|---|---|---|---|
| | Before | After | Before | After | Before | After | Before | After | |
| __ / __ / __ | | | | | | | | | |

| Friday | Breakfast | | Lunch | | Dinner | | Bedtime | | Notes |
|---|---|---|---|---|---|---|---|---|---|
| | Before | After | Before | After | Before | After | Before | After | |
| __ / __ / __ | | | | | | | | | |

| Saturday | Breakfast | | Lunch | | Dinner | | Bedtime | | Notes |
|---|---|---|---|---|---|---|---|---|---|
| | Before | After | Before | After | Before | After | Before | After | |
| __ / __ / __ | | | | | | | | | |

| Sunday | Breakfast | | Lunch | | Dinner | | Bedtime | | Notes |
|---|---|---|---|---|---|---|---|---|---|
| | Before | After | Before | After | Before | After | Before | After | |
| __ / __ / __ | | | | | | | | | |

| Week: _____ | | | | | | | | | Weight: _____ |
|---|---|---|---|---|---|---|---|---|---|

| Monday | Breakfast | | Lunch | | Dinner | | Bedtime | | Notes |
|---|---|---|---|---|---|---|---|---|---|
| | Before | After | Before | After | Before | After | Before | After | |
| __ / __ / __ | | | | | | | | | |

| Tuesday | Breakfast | | Lunch | | Dinner | | Bedtime | | Notes |
|---|---|---|---|---|---|---|---|---|---|
| | Before | After | Before | After | Before | After | Before | After | |
| __ / __ / __ | | | | | | | | | |

| Wednesday | Breakfast | | Lunch | | Dinner | | Bedtime | | Notes |
|---|---|---|---|---|---|---|---|---|---|
| | Before | After | Before | After | Before | After | Before | After | |
| __ / __ / __ | | | | | | | | | |

| Thursday | Breakfast | | Lunch | | Dinner | | Bedtime | | Notes |
|---|---|---|---|---|---|---|---|---|---|
| | Before | After | Before | After | Before | After | Before | After | |
| __ / __ / __ | | | | | | | | | |

| Friday | Breakfast | | Lunch | | Dinner | | Bedtime | | Notes |
|---|---|---|---|---|---|---|---|---|---|
| | Before | After | Before | After | Before | After | Before | After | |
| __ / __ / __ | | | | | | | | | |

| Saturday | Breakfast | | Lunch | | Dinner | | Bedtime | | Notes |
|---|---|---|---|---|---|---|---|---|---|
| | Before | After | Before | After | Before | After | Before | After | |
| __ / __ / __ | | | | | | | | | |

| Sunday | Breakfast | | Lunch | | Dinner | | Bedtime | | Notes |
|---|---|---|---|---|---|---|---|---|---|
| | Before | After | Before | After | Before | After | Before | After | |
| __ / __ / __ | | | | | | | | | |

| Week: _____ | | | | | | | | | Weight: _____ |

| Monday | Breakfast | | Lunch | | Dinner | | Bedtime | | Notes |
|---|---|---|---|---|---|---|---|---|---|
| | Before | After | Before | After | Before | After | Before | After | |
| __/__/__ | | | | | | | | | |

| Tuesday | Breakfast | | Lunch | | Dinner | | Bedtime | | Notes |
|---|---|---|---|---|---|---|---|---|---|
| | Before | After | Before | After | Before | After | Before | After | |
| __/__/__ | | | | | | | | | |

| Wednesday | Breakfast | | Lunch | | Dinner | | Bedtime | | Notes |
|---|---|---|---|---|---|---|---|---|---|
| | Before | After | Before | After | Before | After | Before | After | |
| __/__/__ | | | | | | | | | |

| Thursday | Breakfast | | Lunch | | Dinner | | Bedtime | | Notes |
|---|---|---|---|---|---|---|---|---|---|
| | Before | After | Before | After | Before | After | Before | After | |
| __/__/__ | | | | | | | | | |

| Friday | Breakfast | | Lunch | | Dinner | | Bedtime | | Notes |
|---|---|---|---|---|---|---|---|---|---|
| | Before | After | Before | After | Before | After | Before | After | |
| __/__/__ | | | | | | | | | |

| Saturday | Breakfast | | Lunch | | Dinner | | Bedtime | | Notes |
|---|---|---|---|---|---|---|---|---|---|
| | Before | After | Before | After | Before | After | Before | After | |
| __/__/__ | | | | | | | | | |

| Sunday | Breakfast | | Lunch | | Dinner | | Bedtime | | Notes |
|---|---|---|---|---|---|---|---|---|---|
| | Before | After | Before | After | Before | After | Before | After | |
| __/__/__ | | | | | | | | | |

| Week: _____ | | | | | | | | | Weight: _____ |

| Monday | Breakfast | | Lunch | | Dinner | | Bedtime | | Notes |
|---|---|---|---|---|---|---|---|---|---|
| | Before | After | Before | After | Before | After | Before | After | |
| __ / __ / __ | | | | | | | | | |

| Tuesday | Breakfast | | Lunch | | Dinner | | Bedtime | | Notes |
|---|---|---|---|---|---|---|---|---|---|
| | Before | After | Before | After | Before | After | Before | After | |
| __ / __ / __ | | | | | | | | | |

| Wednesday | Breakfast | | Lunch | | Dinner | | Bedtime | | Notes |
|---|---|---|---|---|---|---|---|---|---|
| | Before | After | Before | After | Before | After | Before | After | |
| __ / __ / __ | | | | | | | | | |

| Thursday | Breakfast | | Lunch | | Dinner | | Bedtime | | Notes |
|---|---|---|---|---|---|---|---|---|---|
| | Before | After | Before | After | Before | After | Before | After | |
| __ / __ / __ | | | | | | | | | |

| Friday | Breakfast | | Lunch | | Dinner | | Bedtime | | Notes |
|---|---|---|---|---|---|---|---|---|---|
| | Before | After | Before | After | Before | After | Before | After | |
| __ / __ / __ | | | | | | | | | |

| Saturday | Breakfast | | Lunch | | Dinner | | Bedtime | | Notes |
|---|---|---|---|---|---|---|---|---|---|
| | Before | After | Before | After | Before | After | Before | After | |
| __ / __ / __ | | | | | | | | | |

| Sunday | Breakfast | | Lunch | | Dinner | | Bedtime | | Notes |
|---|---|---|---|---|---|---|---|---|---|
| | Before | After | Before | After | Before | After | Before | After | |
| __ / __ / __ | | | | | | | | | |

| Week: _____ | | | | | | | | | Weight: _____ |
|---|---|---|---|---|---|---|---|---|---|

| Monday | Breakfast | | Lunch | | Dinner | | Bedtime | | Notes |
|---|---|---|---|---|---|---|---|---|---|
| | Before | After | Before | After | Before | After | Before | After | |
| __ / __ / __ | | | | | | | | | |

| Tuesday | Breakfast | | Lunch | | Dinner | | Bedtime | | Notes |
|---|---|---|---|---|---|---|---|---|---|
| | Before | After | Before | After | Before | After | Before | After | |
| __ / __ / __ | | | | | | | | | |

| Wednesday | Breakfast | | Lunch | | Dinner | | Bedtime | | Notes |
|---|---|---|---|---|---|---|---|---|---|
| | Before | After | Before | After | Before | After | Before | After | |
| __ / __ / __ | | | | | | | | | |

| Thursday | Breakfast | | Lunch | | Dinner | | Bedtime | | Notes |
|---|---|---|---|---|---|---|---|---|---|
| | Before | After | Before | After | Before | After | Before | After | |
| __ / __ / __ | | | | | | | | | |

| Friday | Breakfast | | Lunch | | Dinner | | Bedtime | | Notes |
|---|---|---|---|---|---|---|---|---|---|
| | Before | After | Before | After | Before | After | Before | After | |
| __ / __ / __ | | | | | | | | | |

| Saturday | Breakfast | | Lunch | | Dinner | | Bedtime | | Notes |
|---|---|---|---|---|---|---|---|---|---|
| | Before | After | Before | After | Before | After | Before | After | |
| __ / __ / __ | | | | | | | | | |

| Sunday | Breakfast | | Lunch | | Dinner | | Bedtime | | Notes |
|---|---|---|---|---|---|---|---|---|---|
| | Before | After | Before | After | Before | After | Before | After | |
| __ / __ / __ | | | | | | | | | |

| Week: _____ | | | | | | | | | Weight: _____ |
|---|---|---|---|---|---|---|---|---|---|

| Monday | Breakfast | | Lunch | | Dinner | | Bedtime | | Notes |
|---|---|---|---|---|---|---|---|---|---|
| | Before | After | Before | After | Before | After | Before | After | |
| __ / __ / __ | | | | | | | | | |

| Tuesday | Breakfast | | Lunch | | Dinner | | Bedtime | | Notes |
|---|---|---|---|---|---|---|---|---|---|
| | Before | After | Before | After | Before | After | Before | After | |
| __ / __ / __ | | | | | | | | | |

| Wednesday | Breakfast | | Lunch | | Dinner | | Bedtime | | Notes |
|---|---|---|---|---|---|---|---|---|---|
| | Before | After | Before | After | Before | After | Before | After | |
| __ / __ / __ | | | | | | | | | |

| Thursday | Breakfast | | Lunch | | Dinner | | Bedtime | | Notes |
|---|---|---|---|---|---|---|---|---|---|
| | Before | After | Before | After | Before | After | Before | After | |
| __ / __ / __ | | | | | | | | | |

| Friday | Breakfast | | Lunch | | Dinner | | Bedtime | | Notes |
|---|---|---|---|---|---|---|---|---|---|
| | Before | After | Before | After | Before | After | Before | After | |
| __ / __ / __ | | | | | | | | | |

| Saturday | Breakfast | | Lunch | | Dinner | | Bedtime | | Notes |
|---|---|---|---|---|---|---|---|---|---|
| | Before | After | Before | After | Before | After | Before | After | |
| __ / __ / __ | | | | | | | | | |

| Sunday | Breakfast | | Lunch | | Dinner | | Bedtime | | Notes |
|---|---|---|---|---|---|---|---|---|---|
| | Before | After | Before | After | Before | After | Before | After | |
| __ / __ / __ | | | | | | | | | |

| Week: _____ | | | | | | | | | Weight: _____ |

| Monday | Breakfast | | Lunch | | Dinner | | Bedtime | | Notes |
|---|---|---|---|---|---|---|---|---|---|
| | Before | After | Before | After | Before | After | Before | After | |
| __ / __ / __ | | | | | | | | | |

| Tuesday | Breakfast | | Lunch | | Dinner | | Bedtime | | Notes |
|---|---|---|---|---|---|---|---|---|---|
| | Before | After | Before | After | Before | After | Before | After | |
| __ / __ / __ | | | | | | | | | |

| Wednesday | Breakfast | | Lunch | | Dinner | | Bedtime | | Notes |
|---|---|---|---|---|---|---|---|---|---|
| | Before | After | Before | After | Before | After | Before | After | |
| __ / __ / __ | | | | | | | | | |

| Thursday | Breakfast | | Lunch | | Dinner | | Bedtime | | Notes |
|---|---|---|---|---|---|---|---|---|---|
| | Before | After | Before | After | Before | After | Before | After | |
| __ / __ / __ | | | | | | | | | |

| Friday | Breakfast | | Lunch | | Dinner | | Bedtime | | Notes |
|---|---|---|---|---|---|---|---|---|---|
| | Before | After | Before | After | Before | After | Before | After | |
| __ / __ / __ | | | | | | | | | |

| Saturday | Breakfast | | Lunch | | Dinner | | Bedtime | | Notes |
|---|---|---|---|---|---|---|---|---|---|
| | Before | After | Before | After | Before | After | Before | After | |
| __ / __ / __ | | | | | | | | | |

| Sunday | Breakfast | | Lunch | | Dinner | | Bedtime | | Notes |
|---|---|---|---|---|---|---|---|---|---|
| | Before | After | Before | After | Before | After | Before | After | |
| __ / __ / __ | | | | | | | | | |

| Week: _____ | | | | | | | | | Weight: _____ |
|---|---|---|---|---|---|---|---|---|---|

| Monday | Breakfast | | Lunch | | Dinner | | Bedtime | | Notes |
|---|---|---|---|---|---|---|---|---|---|
| | Before | After | Before | After | Before | After | Before | After | |
| __ / __ / __ | | | | | | | | | |

| Tuesday | Breakfast | | Lunch | | Dinner | | Bedtime | | Notes |
|---|---|---|---|---|---|---|---|---|---|
| | Before | After | Before | After | Before | After | Before | After | |
| __ / __ / __ | | | | | | | | | |

| Wednesday | Breakfast | | Lunch | | Dinner | | Bedtime | | Notes |
|---|---|---|---|---|---|---|---|---|---|
| | Before | After | Before | After | Before | After | Before | After | |
| __ / __ / __ | | | | | | | | | |

| Thursday | Breakfast | | Lunch | | Dinner | | Bedtime | | Notes |
|---|---|---|---|---|---|---|---|---|---|
| | Before | After | Before | After | Before | After | Before | After | |
| __ / __ / __ | | | | | | | | | |

| Friday | Breakfast | | Lunch | | Dinner | | Bedtime | | Notes |
|---|---|---|---|---|---|---|---|---|---|
| | Before | After | Before | After | Before | After | Before | After | |
| __ / __ / __ | | | | | | | | | |

| Saturday | Breakfast | | Lunch | | Dinner | | Bedtime | | Notes |
|---|---|---|---|---|---|---|---|---|---|
| | Before | After | Before | After | Before | After | Before | After | |
| __ / __ / __ | | | | | | | | | |

| Sunday | Breakfast | | Lunch | | Dinner | | Bedtime | | Notes |
|---|---|---|---|---|---|---|---|---|---|
| | Before | After | Before | After | Before | After | Before | After | |
| __ / __ / __ | | | | | | | | | |

| Week: _____ | | | | | | | | | | Weight: _____ |
|---|---|---|---|---|---|---|---|---|---|---|

**Monday**  __/__/__

| | Breakfast | | Lunch | | Dinner | | Bedtime | | Notes |
|---|---|---|---|---|---|---|---|---|---|
| | Before | After | Before | After | Before | After | Before | After | |
| | | | | | | | | | |

**Tuesday**  __/__/__

| | Breakfast | | Lunch | | Dinner | | Bedtime | | Notes |
|---|---|---|---|---|---|---|---|---|---|
| | Before | After | Before | After | Before | After | Before | After | |
| | | | | | | | | | |

**Wednesday**  __/__/__

| | Breakfast | | Lunch | | Dinner | | Bedtime | | Notes |
|---|---|---|---|---|---|---|---|---|---|
| | Before | After | Before | After | Before | After | Before | After | |
| | | | | | | | | | |

**Thursday**  __/__/__

| | Breakfast | | Lunch | | Dinner | | Bedtime | | Notes |
|---|---|---|---|---|---|---|---|---|---|
| | Before | After | Before | After | Before | After | Before | After | |
| | | | | | | | | | |

**Friday**  __/__/__

| | Breakfast | | Lunch | | Dinner | | Bedtime | | Notes |
|---|---|---|---|---|---|---|---|---|---|
| | Before | After | Before | After | Before | After | Before | After | |
| | | | | | | | | | |

**Saturday**  __/__/__

| | Breakfast | | Lunch | | Dinner | | Bedtime | | Notes |
|---|---|---|---|---|---|---|---|---|---|
| | Before | After | Before | After | Before | After | Before | After | |
| | | | | | | | | | |

**Sunday**  __/__/__

| | Breakfast | | Lunch | | Dinner | | Bedtime | | Notes |
|---|---|---|---|---|---|---|---|---|---|
| | Before | After | Before | After | Before | After | Before | After | |
| | | | | | | | | | |

| Week: _____ | | | | | | | | Weight: _____ | |
|---|---|---|---|---|---|---|---|---|---|

| Monday | Breakfast | | Lunch | | Dinner | | Bedtime | | Notes |
|---|---|---|---|---|---|---|---|---|---|
| | Before | After | Before | After | Before | After | Before | After | |
| __ / __ / __ | | | | | | | | | |

| Tuesday | Breakfast | | Lunch | | Dinner | | Bedtime | | Notes |
|---|---|---|---|---|---|---|---|---|---|
| | Before | After | Before | After | Before | After | Before | After | |
| __ / __ / __ | | | | | | | | | |

| Wednesday | Breakfast | | Lunch | | Dinner | | Bedtime | | Notes |
|---|---|---|---|---|---|---|---|---|---|
| | Before | After | Before | After | Before | After | Before | After | |
| __ / __ / __ | | | | | | | | | |

| Thursday | Breakfast | | Lunch | | Dinner | | Bedtime | | Notes |
|---|---|---|---|---|---|---|---|---|---|
| | Before | After | Before | After | Before | After | Before | After | |
| __ / __ / __ | | | | | | | | | |

| Friday | Breakfast | | Lunch | | Dinner | | Bedtime | | Notes |
|---|---|---|---|---|---|---|---|---|---|
| | Before | After | Before | After | Before | After | Before | After | |
| __ / __ / __ | | | | | | | | | |

| Saturday | Breakfast | | Lunch | | Dinner | | Bedtime | | Notes |
|---|---|---|---|---|---|---|---|---|---|
| | Before | After | Before | After | Before | After | Before | After | |
| __ / __ / __ | | | | | | | | | |

| Sunday | Breakfast | | Lunch | | Dinner | | Bedtime | | Notes |
|---|---|---|---|---|---|---|---|---|---|
| | Before | After | Before | After | Before | After | Before | After | |
| __ / __ / __ | | | | | | | | | |

| Monday | Breakfast | | Lunch | | Dinner | | Bedtime | | Notes |
|---|---|---|---|---|---|---|---|---|---|
| | Before | After | Before | After | Before | After | Before | After | |
| __/__/__ | | | | | | | | | |

| Tuesday | Breakfast | | Lunch | | Dinner | | Bedtime | | Notes |
|---|---|---|---|---|---|---|---|---|---|
| | Before | After | Before | After | Before | After | Before | After | |
| __/__/__ | | | | | | | | | |

| Wednesday | Breakfast | | Lunch | | Dinner | | Bedtime | | Notes |
|---|---|---|---|---|---|---|---|---|---|
| | Before | After | Before | After | Before | After | Before | After | |
| __/__/__ | | | | | | | | | |

| Thursday | Breakfast | | Lunch | | Dinner | | Bedtime | | Notes |
|---|---|---|---|---|---|---|---|---|---|
| | Before | After | Before | After | Before | After | Before | After | |
| __/__/__ | | | | | | | | | |

| Friday | Breakfast | | Lunch | | Dinner | | Bedtime | | Notes |
|---|---|---|---|---|---|---|---|---|---|
| | Before | After | Before | After | Before | After | Before | After | |
| __/__/__ | | | | | | | | | |

| Saturday | Breakfast | | Lunch | | Dinner | | Bedtime | | Notes |
|---|---|---|---|---|---|---|---|---|---|
| | Before | After | Before | After | Before | After | Before | After | |
| __/__/__ | | | | | | | | | |

| Sunday | Breakfast | | Lunch | | Dinner | | Bedtime | | Notes |
|---|---|---|---|---|---|---|---|---|---|
| | Before | After | Before | After | Before | After | Before | After | |
| __/__/__ | | | | | | | | | |

| Week: _____ | | | | | | | | | Weight: _____ |
|---|---|---|---|---|---|---|---|---|---|

| Monday | Breakfast | | Lunch | | Dinner | | Bedtime | | Notes |
|---|---|---|---|---|---|---|---|---|---|
| | Before | After | Before | After | Before | After | Before | After | |
| __ / __ / __ | | | | | | | | | |

| Tuesday | Breakfast | | Lunch | | Dinner | | Bedtime | | Notes |
|---|---|---|---|---|---|---|---|---|---|
| | Before | After | Before | After | Before | After | Before | After | |
| __ / __ / __ | | | | | | | | | |

| Wednesday | Breakfast | | Lunch | | Dinner | | Bedtime | | Notes |
|---|---|---|---|---|---|---|---|---|---|
| | Before | After | Before | After | Before | After | Before | After | |
| __ / __ / __ | | | | | | | | | |

| Thursday | Breakfast | | Lunch | | Dinner | | Bedtime | | Notes |
|---|---|---|---|---|---|---|---|---|---|
| | Before | After | Before | After | Before | After | Before | After | |
| __ / __ / __ | | | | | | | | | |

| Friday | Breakfast | | Lunch | | Dinner | | Bedtime | | Notes |
|---|---|---|---|---|---|---|---|---|---|
| | Before | After | Before | After | Before | After | Before | After | |
| __ / __ / __ | | | | | | | | | |

| Saturday | Breakfast | | Lunch | | Dinner | | Bedtime | | Notes |
|---|---|---|---|---|---|---|---|---|---|
| | Before | After | Before | After | Before | After | Before | After | |
| __ / __ / __ | | | | | | | | | |

| Sunday | Breakfast | | Lunch | | Dinner | | Bedtime | | Notes |
|---|---|---|---|---|---|---|---|---|---|
| | Before | After | Before | After | Before | After | Before | After | |
| __ / __ / __ | | | | | | | | | |

| Week: _____ | | | | | | | | | Weight: _____ |
|---|---|---|---|---|---|---|---|---|---|

| Monday | Breakfast | | Lunch | | Dinner | | Bedtime | | Notes |
|---|---|---|---|---|---|---|---|---|---|
| | Before | After | Before | After | Before | After | Before | After | |
| __ / __ / __ | | | | | | | | | |

| Tuesday | Breakfast | | Lunch | | Dinner | | Bedtime | | Notes |
|---|---|---|---|---|---|---|---|---|---|
| | Before | After | Before | After | Before | After | Before | After | |
| __ / __ / __ | | | | | | | | | |

| Wednesday | Breakfast | | Lunch | | Dinner | | Bedtime | | Notes |
|---|---|---|---|---|---|---|---|---|---|
| | Before | After | Before | After | Before | After | Before | After | |
| __ / __ / __ | | | | | | | | | |

| Thursday | Breakfast | | Lunch | | Dinner | | Bedtime | | Notes |
|---|---|---|---|---|---|---|---|---|---|
| | Before | After | Before | After | Before | After | Before | After | |
| __ / __ / __ | | | | | | | | | |

| Friday | Breakfast | | Lunch | | Dinner | | Bedtime | | Notes |
|---|---|---|---|---|---|---|---|---|---|
| | Before | After | Before | After | Before | After | Before | After | |
| __ / __ / __ | | | | | | | | | |

| Saturday | Breakfast | | Lunch | | Dinner | | Bedtime | | Notes |
|---|---|---|---|---|---|---|---|---|---|
| | Before | After | Before | After | Before | After | Before | After | |
| __ / __ / __ | | | | | | | | | |

| Sunday | Breakfast | | Lunch | | Dinner | | Bedtime | | Notes |
|---|---|---|---|---|---|---|---|---|---|
| | Before | After | Before | After | Before | After | Before | After | |
| __ / __ / __ | | | | | | | | | |

| Week: _____ | | | | | | | | | Weight: _____ |
|---|---|---|---|---|---|---|---|---|---|

| Monday | Breakfast | | Lunch | | Dinner | | Bedtime | | Notes |
|---|---|---|---|---|---|---|---|---|---|
| | Before | After | Before | After | Before | After | Before | After | |
| __ / __ / __ | | | | | | | | | |

| Tuesday | Breakfast | | Lunch | | Dinner | | Bedtime | | Notes |
|---|---|---|---|---|---|---|---|---|---|
| | Before | After | Before | After | Before | After | Before | After | |
| __ / __ / __ | | | | | | | | | |

| Wednesday | Breakfast | | Lunch | | Dinner | | Bedtime | | Notes |
|---|---|---|---|---|---|---|---|---|---|
| | Before | After | Before | After | Before | After | Before | After | |
| __ / __ / __ | | | | | | | | | |

| Thursday | Breakfast | | Lunch | | Dinner | | Bedtime | | Notes |
|---|---|---|---|---|---|---|---|---|---|
| | Before | After | Before | After | Before | After | Before | After | |
| __ / __ / __ | | | | | | | | | |

| Friday | Breakfast | | Lunch | | Dinner | | Bedtime | | Notes |
|---|---|---|---|---|---|---|---|---|---|
| | Before | After | Before | After | Before | After | Before | After | |
| __ / __ / __ | | | | | | | | | |

| Saturday | Breakfast | | Lunch | | Dinner | | Bedtime | | Notes |
|---|---|---|---|---|---|---|---|---|---|
| | Before | After | Before | After | Before | After | Before | After | |
| __ / __ / __ | | | | | | | | | |

| Sunday | Breakfast | | Lunch | | Dinner | | Bedtime | | Notes |
|---|---|---|---|---|---|---|---|---|---|
| | Before | After | Before | After | Before | After | Before | After | |
| __ / __ / __ | | | | | | | | | |

| Week: _____ | | | | | | | | | Weight: _____ |
|---|---|---|---|---|---|---|---|---|---|

| Monday | Breakfast | | Lunch | | Dinner | | Bedtime | | Notes |
|---|---|---|---|---|---|---|---|---|---|
| | Before | After | Before | After | Before | After | Before | After | |
| __ / __ / __ | | | | | | | | | |

| Tuesday | Breakfast | | Lunch | | Dinner | | Bedtime | | Notes |
|---|---|---|---|---|---|---|---|---|---|
| | Before | After | Before | After | Before | After | Before | After | |
| __ / __ / __ | | | | | | | | | |

| Wednesday | Breakfast | | Lunch | | Dinner | | Bedtime | | Notes |
|---|---|---|---|---|---|---|---|---|---|
| | Before | After | Before | After | Before | After | Before | After | |
| __ / __ / __ | | | | | | | | | |

| Thursday | Breakfast | | Lunch | | Dinner | | Bedtime | | Notes |
|---|---|---|---|---|---|---|---|---|---|
| | Before | After | Before | After | Before | After | Before | After | |
| __ / __ / __ | | | | | | | | | |

| Friday | Breakfast | | Lunch | | Dinner | | Bedtime | | Notes |
|---|---|---|---|---|---|---|---|---|---|
| | Before | After | Before | After | Before | After | Before | After | |
| __ / __ / __ | | | | | | | | | |

| Saturday | Breakfast | | Lunch | | Dinner | | Bedtime | | Notes |
|---|---|---|---|---|---|---|---|---|---|
| | Before | After | Before | After | Before | After | Before | After | |
| __ / __ / __ | | | | | | | | | |

| Sunday | Breakfast | | Lunch | | Dinner | | Bedtime | | Notes |
|---|---|---|---|---|---|---|---|---|---|
| | Before | After | Before | After | Before | After | Before | After | |
| __ / __ / __ | | | | | | | | | |

| Week: _____ | | | | | | | | | Weight: _____ |

| Monday | Breakfast | | Lunch | | Dinner | | Bedtime | | Notes |
|---|---|---|---|---|---|---|---|---|---|
| | Before | After | Before | After | Before | After | Before | After | |
| __/__/__ | | | | | | | | | |

| Tuesday | Breakfast | | Lunch | | Dinner | | Bedtime | | Notes |
|---|---|---|---|---|---|---|---|---|---|
| | Before | After | Before | After | Before | After | Before | After | |
| __/__/__ | | | | | | | | | |

| Wednesday | Breakfast | | Lunch | | Dinner | | Bedtime | | Notes |
|---|---|---|---|---|---|---|---|---|---|
| | Before | After | Before | After | Before | After | Before | After | |
| __/__/__ | | | | | | | | | |

| Thursday | Breakfast | | Lunch | | Dinner | | Bedtime | | Notes |
|---|---|---|---|---|---|---|---|---|---|
| | Before | After | Before | After | Before | After | Before | After | |
| __/__/__ | | | | | | | | | |

| Friday | Breakfast | | Lunch | | Dinner | | Bedtime | | Notes |
|---|---|---|---|---|---|---|---|---|---|
| | Before | After | Before | After | Before | After | Before | After | |
| __/__/__ | | | | | | | | | |

| Saturday | Breakfast | | Lunch | | Dinner | | Bedtime | | Notes |
|---|---|---|---|---|---|---|---|---|---|
| | Before | After | Before | After | Before | After | Before | After | |
| __/__/__ | | | | | | | | | |

| Sunday | Breakfast | | Lunch | | Dinner | | Bedtime | | Notes |
|---|---|---|---|---|---|---|---|---|---|
| | Before | After | Before | After | Before | After | Before | After | |
| __/__/__ | | | | | | | | | |

| Week: _____ | | | | | | | | | Weight: _____ |
|---|---|---|---|---|---|---|---|---|---|

| Monday | Breakfast | | Lunch | | Dinner | | Bedtime | | Notes |
|---|---|---|---|---|---|---|---|---|---|
| | Before | After | Before | After | Before | After | Before | After | |
| __/__/__ | | | | | | | | | |

| Tuesday | Breakfast | | Lunch | | Dinner | | Bedtime | | Notes |
|---|---|---|---|---|---|---|---|---|---|
| | Before | After | Before | After | Before | After | Before | After | |
| __/__/__ | | | | | | | | | |

| Wednesday | Breakfast | | Lunch | | Dinner | | Bedtime | | Notes |
|---|---|---|---|---|---|---|---|---|---|
| | Before | After | Before | After | Before | After | Before | After | |
| __/__/__ | | | | | | | | | |

| Thursday | Breakfast | | Lunch | | Dinner | | Bedtime | | Notes |
|---|---|---|---|---|---|---|---|---|---|
| | Before | After | Before | After | Before | After | Before | After | |
| __/__/__ | | | | | | | | | |

| Friday | Breakfast | | Lunch | | Dinner | | Bedtime | | Notes |
|---|---|---|---|---|---|---|---|---|---|
| | Before | After | Before | After | Before | After | Before | After | |
| __/__/__ | | | | | | | | | |

| Saturday | Breakfast | | Lunch | | Dinner | | Bedtime | | Notes |
|---|---|---|---|---|---|---|---|---|---|
| | Before | After | Before | After | Before | After | Before | After | |
| __/__/__ | | | | | | | | | |

| Sunday | Breakfast | | Lunch | | Dinner | | Bedtime | | Notes |
|---|---|---|---|---|---|---|---|---|---|
| | Before | After | Before | After | Before | After | Before | After | |
| __/__/__ | | | | | | | | | |

| Week: _____ | | | | | | | | | Weight: _____ |

| Monday | Breakfast | | Lunch | | Dinner | | Bedtime | | Notes |
|---|---|---|---|---|---|---|---|---|---|
| | Before | After | Before | After | Before | After | Before | After | |
| __ / __ / __ | | | | | | | | | |

| Tuesday | Breakfast | | Lunch | | Dinner | | Bedtime | | Notes |
|---|---|---|---|---|---|---|---|---|---|
| | Before | After | Before | After | Before | After | Before | After | |
| __ / __ / __ | | | | | | | | | |

| Wednesday | Breakfast | | Lunch | | Dinner | | Bedtime | | Notes |
|---|---|---|---|---|---|---|---|---|---|
| | Before | After | Before | After | Before | After | Before | After | |
| __ / __ / __ | | | | | | | | | |

| Thursday | Breakfast | | Lunch | | Dinner | | Bedtime | | Notes |
|---|---|---|---|---|---|---|---|---|---|
| | Before | After | Before | After | Before | After | Before | After | |
| __ / __ / __ | | | | | | | | | |

| Friday | Breakfast | | Lunch | | Dinner | | Bedtime | | Notes |
|---|---|---|---|---|---|---|---|---|---|
| | Before | After | Before | After | Before | After | Before | After | |
| __ / __ / __ | | | | | | | | | |

| Saturday | Breakfast | | Lunch | | Dinner | | Bedtime | | Notes |
|---|---|---|---|---|---|---|---|---|---|
| | Before | After | Before | After | Before | After | Before | After | |
| __ / __ / __ | | | | | | | | | |

| Sunday | Breakfast | | Lunch | | Dinner | | Bedtime | | Notes |
|---|---|---|---|---|---|---|---|---|---|
| | Before | After | Before | After | Before | After | Before | After | |
| __ / __ / __ | | | | | | | | | |

| Monday | Breakfast | | Lunch | | Dinner | | Bedtime | | Notes |
|---|---|---|---|---|---|---|---|---|---|
| | Before | After | Before | After | Before | After | Before | After | |
| __ / __ / __ | | | | | | | | | |

| Tuesday | Breakfast | | Lunch | | Dinner | | Bedtime | | Notes |
|---|---|---|---|---|---|---|---|---|---|
| | Before | After | Before | After | Before | After | Before | After | |
| __ / __ / __ | | | | | | | | | |

| Wednesday | Breakfast | | Lunch | | Dinner | | Bedtime | | Notes |
|---|---|---|---|---|---|---|---|---|---|
| | Before | After | Before | After | Before | After | Before | After | |
| __ / __ / __ | | | | | | | | | |

| Thursday | Breakfast | | Lunch | | Dinner | | Bedtime | | Notes |
|---|---|---|---|---|---|---|---|---|---|
| | Before | After | Before | After | Before | After | Before | After | |
| __ / __ / __ | | | | | | | | | |

| Friday | Breakfast | | Lunch | | Dinner | | Bedtime | | Notes |
|---|---|---|---|---|---|---|---|---|---|
| | Before | After | Before | After | Before | After | Before | After | |
| __ / __ / __ | | | | | | | | | |

| Saturday | Breakfast | | Lunch | | Dinner | | Bedtime | | Notes |
|---|---|---|---|---|---|---|---|---|---|
| | Before | After | Before | After | Before | After | Before | After | |
| __ / __ / __ | | | | | | | | | |

| Sunday | Breakfast | | Lunch | | Dinner | | Bedtime | | Notes |
|---|---|---|---|---|---|---|---|---|---|
| | Before | After | Before | After | Before | After | Before | After | |
| __ / __ / __ | | | | | | | | | |

Week: _____        Weight: _____

| Monday __/__/__ | Breakfast | | Lunch | | Dinner | | Bedtime | | Notes |
|---|---|---|---|---|---|---|---|---|---|
| | Before | After | Before | After | Before | After | Before | After | |
| | | | | | | | | | |

| Tuesday __/__/__ | Breakfast | | Lunch | | Dinner | | Bedtime | | Notes |
|---|---|---|---|---|---|---|---|---|---|
| | Before | After | Before | After | Before | After | Before | After | |
| | | | | | | | | | |

| Wednesday __/__/__ | Breakfast | | Lunch | | Dinner | | Bedtime | | Notes |
|---|---|---|---|---|---|---|---|---|---|
| | Before | After | Before | After | Before | After | Before | After | |
| | | | | | | | | | |

| Thursday __/__/__ | Breakfast | | Lunch | | Dinner | | Bedtime | | Notes |
|---|---|---|---|---|---|---|---|---|---|
| | Before | After | Before | After | Before | After | Before | After | |
| | | | | | | | | | |

| Friday __/__/__ | Breakfast | | Lunch | | Dinner | | Bedtime | | Notes |
|---|---|---|---|---|---|---|---|---|---|
| | Before | After | Before | After | Before | After | Before | After | |
| | | | | | | | | | |

| Saturday __/__/__ | Breakfast | | Lunch | | Dinner | | Bedtime | | Notes |
|---|---|---|---|---|---|---|---|---|---|
| | Before | After | Before | After | Before | After | Before | After | |
| | | | | | | | | | |

| Sunday __/__/__ | Breakfast | | Lunch | | Dinner | | Bedtime | | Notes |
|---|---|---|---|---|---|---|---|---|---|
| | Before | After | Before | After | Before | After | Before | After | |
| | | | | | | | | | |

| Week: _____ | | | | | | | | | Weight: _____ |
|---|---|---|---|---|---|---|---|---|---|

| Monday | Breakfast | | Lunch | | Dinner | | Bedtime | | Notes |
|---|---|---|---|---|---|---|---|---|---|
| | Before | After | Before | After | Before | After | Before | After | |
| __ / __ / __ | | | | | | | | | |

| Tuesday | Breakfast | | Lunch | | Dinner | | Bedtime | | Notes |
|---|---|---|---|---|---|---|---|---|---|
| | Before | After | Before | After | Before | After | Before | After | |
| __ / __ / __ | | | | | | | | | |

| Wednesday | Breakfast | | Lunch | | Dinner | | Bedtime | | Notes |
|---|---|---|---|---|---|---|---|---|---|
| | Before | After | Before | After | Before | After | Before | After | |
| __ / __ / __ | | | | | | | | | |

| Thursday | Breakfast | | Lunch | | Dinner | | Bedtime | | Notes |
|---|---|---|---|---|---|---|---|---|---|
| | Before | After | Before | After | Before | After | Before | After | |
| __ / __ / __ | | | | | | | | | |

| Friday | Breakfast | | Lunch | | Dinner | | Bedtime | | Notes |
|---|---|---|---|---|---|---|---|---|---|
| | Before | After | Before | After | Before | After | Before | After | |
| __ / __ / __ | | | | | | | | | |

| Saturday | Breakfast | | Lunch | | Dinner | | Bedtime | | Notes |
|---|---|---|---|---|---|---|---|---|---|
| | Before | After | Before | After | Before | After | Before | After | |
| __ / __ / __ | | | | | | | | | |

| Sunday | Breakfast | | Lunch | | Dinner | | Bedtime | | Notes |
|---|---|---|---|---|---|---|---|---|---|
| | Before | After | Before | After | Before | After | Before | After | |
| __ / __ / __ | | | | | | | | | |

| Week: _____ | | | | | | | | | Weight: _____ |

| Monday | Breakfast | | Lunch | | Dinner | | Bedtime | | Notes |
|---|---|---|---|---|---|---|---|---|---|
| | Before | After | Before | After | Before | After | Before | After | |
| __ / __ / __ | | | | | | | | | |

| Tuesday | Breakfast | | Lunch | | Dinner | | Bedtime | | Notes |
|---|---|---|---|---|---|---|---|---|---|
| | Before | After | Before | After | Before | After | Before | After | |
| __ / __ / __ | | | | | | | | | |

| Wednesday | Breakfast | | Lunch | | Dinner | | Bedtime | | Notes |
|---|---|---|---|---|---|---|---|---|---|
| | Before | After | Before | After | Before | After | Before | After | |
| __ / __ / __ | | | | | | | | | |

| Thursday | Breakfast | | Lunch | | Dinner | | Bedtime | | Notes |
|---|---|---|---|---|---|---|---|---|---|
| | Before | After | Before | After | Before | After | Before | After | |
| __ / __ / __ | | | | | | | | | |

| Friday | Breakfast | | Lunch | | Dinner | | Bedtime | | Notes |
|---|---|---|---|---|---|---|---|---|---|
| | Before | After | Before | After | Before | After | Before | After | |
| __ / __ / __ | | | | | | | | | |

| Saturday | Breakfast | | Lunch | | Dinner | | Bedtime | | Notes |
|---|---|---|---|---|---|---|---|---|---|
| | Before | After | Before | After | Before | After | Before | After | |
| __ / __ / __ | | | | | | | | | |

| Sunday | Breakfast | | Lunch | | Dinner | | Bedtime | | Notes |
|---|---|---|---|---|---|---|---|---|---|
| | Before | After | Before | After | Before | After | Before | After | |
| __ / __ / __ | | | | | | | | | |

| Week: _____ | | | | | | | | | Weight: _____ |
|---|---|---|---|---|---|---|---|---|---|

| Monday | Breakfast | | Lunch | | Dinner | | Bedtime | | Notes |
|---|---|---|---|---|---|---|---|---|---|
| | Before | After | Before | After | Before | After | Before | After | |
| __ / __ / __ | | | | | | | | | |

| Tuesday | Breakfast | | Lunch | | Dinner | | Bedtime | | Notes |
|---|---|---|---|---|---|---|---|---|---|
| | Before | After | Before | After | Before | After | Before | After | |
| __ / __ / __ | | | | | | | | | |

| Wednesday | Breakfast | | Lunch | | Dinner | | Bedtime | | Notes |
|---|---|---|---|---|---|---|---|---|---|
| | Before | After | Before | After | Before | After | Before | After | |
| __ / __ / __ | | | | | | | | | |

| Thursday | Breakfast | | Lunch | | Dinner | | Bedtime | | Notes |
|---|---|---|---|---|---|---|---|---|---|
| | Before | After | Before | After | Before | After | Before | After | |
| __ / __ / __ | | | | | | | | | |

| Friday | Breakfast | | Lunch | | Dinner | | Bedtime | | Notes |
|---|---|---|---|---|---|---|---|---|---|
| | Before | After | Before | After | Before | After | Before | After | |
| __ / __ / __ | | | | | | | | | |

| Saturday | Breakfast | | Lunch | | Dinner | | Bedtime | | Notes |
|---|---|---|---|---|---|---|---|---|---|
| | Before | After | Before | After | Before | After | Before | After | |
| __ / __ / __ | | | | | | | | | |

| Sunday | Breakfast | | Lunch | | Dinner | | Bedtime | | Notes |
|---|---|---|---|---|---|---|---|---|---|
| | Before | After | Before | After | Before | After | Before | After | |
| __ / __ / __ | | | | | | | | | |

| Monday | Breakfast | | Lunch | | Dinner | | Bedtime | | Notes |
|---|---|---|---|---|---|---|---|---|---|
| | Before | After | Before | After | Before | After | Before | After | |
| __ / __ / __ | | | | | | | | | |

| Tuesday | Breakfast | | Lunch | | Dinner | | Bedtime | | Notes |
|---|---|---|---|---|---|---|---|---|---|
| | Before | After | Before | After | Before | After | Before | After | |
| __ / __ / __ | | | | | | | | | |

| Wednesday | Breakfast | | Lunch | | Dinner | | Bedtime | | Notes |
|---|---|---|---|---|---|---|---|---|---|
| | Before | After | Before | After | Before | After | Before | After | |
| __ / __ / __ | | | | | | | | | |

| Thursday | Breakfast | | Lunch | | Dinner | | Bedtime | | Notes |
|---|---|---|---|---|---|---|---|---|---|
| | Before | After | Before | After | Before | After | Before | After | |
| __ / __ / __ | | | | | | | | | |

| Friday | Breakfast | | Lunch | | Dinner | | Bedtime | | Notes |
|---|---|---|---|---|---|---|---|---|---|
| | Before | After | Before | After | Before | After | Before | After | |
| __ / __ / __ | | | | | | | | | |

| Saturday | Breakfast | | Lunch | | Dinner | | Bedtime | | Notes |
|---|---|---|---|---|---|---|---|---|---|
| | Before | After | Before | After | Before | After | Before | After | |
| __ / __ / __ | | | | | | | | | |

| Sunday | Breakfast | | Lunch | | Dinner | | Bedtime | | Notes |
|---|---|---|---|---|---|---|---|---|---|
| | Before | After | Before | After | Before | After | Before | After | |
| __ / __ / __ | | | | | | | | | |

| Week: _____ | | | | | | | | | Weight: _____ |

| Monday | Breakfast | | Lunch | | Dinner | | Bedtime | | Notes |
|---|---|---|---|---|---|---|---|---|---|
| | Before | After | Before | After | Before | After | Before | After | |
| __/__/__ | | | | | | | | | |

| Tuesday | Breakfast | | Lunch | | Dinner | | Bedtime | | Notes |
|---|---|---|---|---|---|---|---|---|---|
| | Before | After | Before | After | Before | After | Before | After | |
| __/__/__ | | | | | | | | | |

| Wednesday | Breakfast | | Lunch | | Dinner | | Bedtime | | Notes |
|---|---|---|---|---|---|---|---|---|---|
| | Before | After | Before | After | Before | After | Before | After | |
| __/__/__ | | | | | | | | | |

| Thursday | Breakfast | | Lunch | | Dinner | | Bedtime | | Notes |
|---|---|---|---|---|---|---|---|---|---|
| | Before | After | Before | After | Before | After | Before | After | |
| __/__/__ | | | | | | | | | |

| Friday | Breakfast | | Lunch | | Dinner | | Bedtime | | Notes |
|---|---|---|---|---|---|---|---|---|---|
| | Before | After | Before | After | Before | After | Before | After | |
| __/__/__ | | | | | | | | | |

| Saturday | Breakfast | | Lunch | | Dinner | | Bedtime | | Notes |
|---|---|---|---|---|---|---|---|---|---|
| | Before | After | Before | After | Before | After | Before | After | |
| __/__/__ | | | | | | | | | |

| Sunday | Breakfast | | Lunch | | Dinner | | Bedtime | | Notes |
|---|---|---|---|---|---|---|---|---|---|
| | Before | After | Before | After | Before | After | Before | After | |
| __/__/__ | | | | | | | | | |

| Monday __/__/__ | Breakfast | | Lunch | | Dinner | | Bedtime | | Notes |
|---|---|---|---|---|---|---|---|---|---|
| | Before | After | Before | After | Before | After | Before | After | |
| | | | | | | | | | |

| Tuesday __/__/__ | Breakfast | | Lunch | | Dinner | | Bedtime | | Notes |
|---|---|---|---|---|---|---|---|---|---|
| | Before | After | Before | After | Before | After | Before | After | |
| | | | | | | | | | |

| Wednesday __/__/__ | Breakfast | | Lunch | | Dinner | | Bedtime | | Notes |
|---|---|---|---|---|---|---|---|---|---|
| | Before | After | Before | After | Before | After | Before | After | |
| | | | | | | | | | |

| Thursday __/__/__ | Breakfast | | Lunch | | Dinner | | Bedtime | | Notes |
|---|---|---|---|---|---|---|---|---|---|
| | Before | After | Before | After | Before | After | Before | After | |
| | | | | | | | | | |

| Friday __/__/__ | Breakfast | | Lunch | | Dinner | | Bedtime | | Notes |
|---|---|---|---|---|---|---|---|---|---|
| | Before | After | Before | After | Before | After | Before | After | |
| | | | | | | | | | |

| Saturday __/__/__ | Breakfast | | Lunch | | Dinner | | Bedtime | | Notes |
|---|---|---|---|---|---|---|---|---|---|
| | Before | After | Before | After | Before | After | Before | After | |
| | | | | | | | | | |

| Sunday __/__/__ | Breakfast | | Lunch | | Dinner | | Bedtime | | Notes |
|---|---|---|---|---|---|---|---|---|---|
| | Before | After | Before | After | Before | After | Before | After | |
| | | | | | | | | | |

| Week: _____ | | | | | | | | | Weight: _____ |
|---|---|---|---|---|---|---|---|---|---|

| Monday | Breakfast | | Lunch | | Dinner | | Bedtime | | Notes |
|---|---|---|---|---|---|---|---|---|---|
| | Before | After | Before | After | Before | After | Before | After | |
| __ / __ / __ | | | | | | | | | |

| Tuesday | Breakfast | | Lunch | | Dinner | | Bedtime | | Notes |
|---|---|---|---|---|---|---|---|---|---|
| | Before | After | Before | After | Before | After | Before | After | |
| __ / __ / __ | | | | | | | | | |

| Wednesday | Breakfast | | Lunch | | Dinner | | Bedtime | | Notes |
|---|---|---|---|---|---|---|---|---|---|
| | Before | After | Before | After | Before | After | Before | After | |
| __ / __ / __ | | | | | | | | | |

| Thursday | Breakfast | | Lunch | | Dinner | | Bedtime | | Notes |
|---|---|---|---|---|---|---|---|---|---|
| | Before | After | Before | After | Before | After | Before | After | |
| __ / __ / __ | | | | | | | | | |

| Friday | Breakfast | | Lunch | | Dinner | | Bedtime | | Notes |
|---|---|---|---|---|---|---|---|---|---|
| | Before | After | Before | After | Before | After | Before | After | |
| __ / __ / __ | | | | | | | | | |

| Saturday | Breakfast | | Lunch | | Dinner | | Bedtime | | Notes |
|---|---|---|---|---|---|---|---|---|---|
| | Before | After | Before | After | Before | After | Before | After | |
| __ / __ / __ | | | | | | | | | |

| Sunday | Breakfast | | Lunch | | Dinner | | Bedtime | | Notes |
|---|---|---|---|---|---|---|---|---|---|
| | Before | After | Before | After | Before | After | Before | After | |
| __ / __ / __ | | | | | | | | | |

Made in United States
Troutdale, OR
03/21/2024

18639118R00060